Nature's Secret Weight Loss for Beginners in 2023

A healthy collection And scientific proven Approach to reduce stubborn belly fat, Achieve weight loss and Stay healthy

BY

Janet R. Sheppard

Copyright

© 2023 Janet R. Sheppard

Disclaimer

This book, "Nature's Secret Weight Loss for Beginners in 2023," contains information that is solely meant to be used for general educational reasons. It is not intended to replace expert medical guidance, diagnosis, or care. When in doubt about a medical problem, never hesitate to consult your doctor or another trained healthcare professional.

The publisher and author of this book disclaim all liability for any special health or allergy needs that may call for medical supervision. They also disclaim all liability for any harm that may result from any preparation, action, treatment, or outcome for anyone who reads or uses the information in this book. The references are given purely for informative purposes and do not imply any support for any websites or other sources.

You assume complete responsibility for any action you take based on the information in this book. Any external websites that are linked to from this book are not under the control of the author or publisher.

You accept the terms and conditions stated in this disclaimer by reading this book.

About the Author

Janet R. Sheppard is a passionate advocate for health and well-being, dedicated to inspiring others to embrace a balanced and vibrant lifestyle. With a profound interest in holistic health practices, she has become a trusted voice in the realm of healthy living.

Janet's journey into the world of health and well-being began as a personal quest for vitality and balance. Her experiences and studies have culminated in a wealth of knowledge, empowering her to guide others on their own paths to optimal health.

Embracing a holistic approach to health, Janet emphasizes the integration of physical, mental, and emotional well-being. She believes that true vitality arises from nurturing the body, mind, and spirit in harmony. Her teachings and insights reflect this comprehensive perspective, offering practical advice and transformative practices.

As a happily married individual, Janet understands the unique challenges and opportunities that come with nurturing a shared commitment to well-being within a partnership. She believes that a supportive and health-conscious relationship can be a cornerstone for personal growth and mutual fulfillment.

Beyond her dedication to health advocacy, Janet cherishes quality time spent with her loved ones, immersing herself in nature, and exploring new avenues for personal growth. Her own life serves as a testament to the transformative power of embracing a health-conscious lifestyle.

TABLE OF CONTENT

SMART SNACKING

Eating Mindfully

Tracking Your Food Intake

Getting Enough Sleep

Exercising More Often

Guidance for Making Sustainable Lifestyle Changes

Tracking Your Progress

Conclusion
Reflecting on Your Journey and Looking Ahead
Encouragement and Final Words of Advice

Appendices

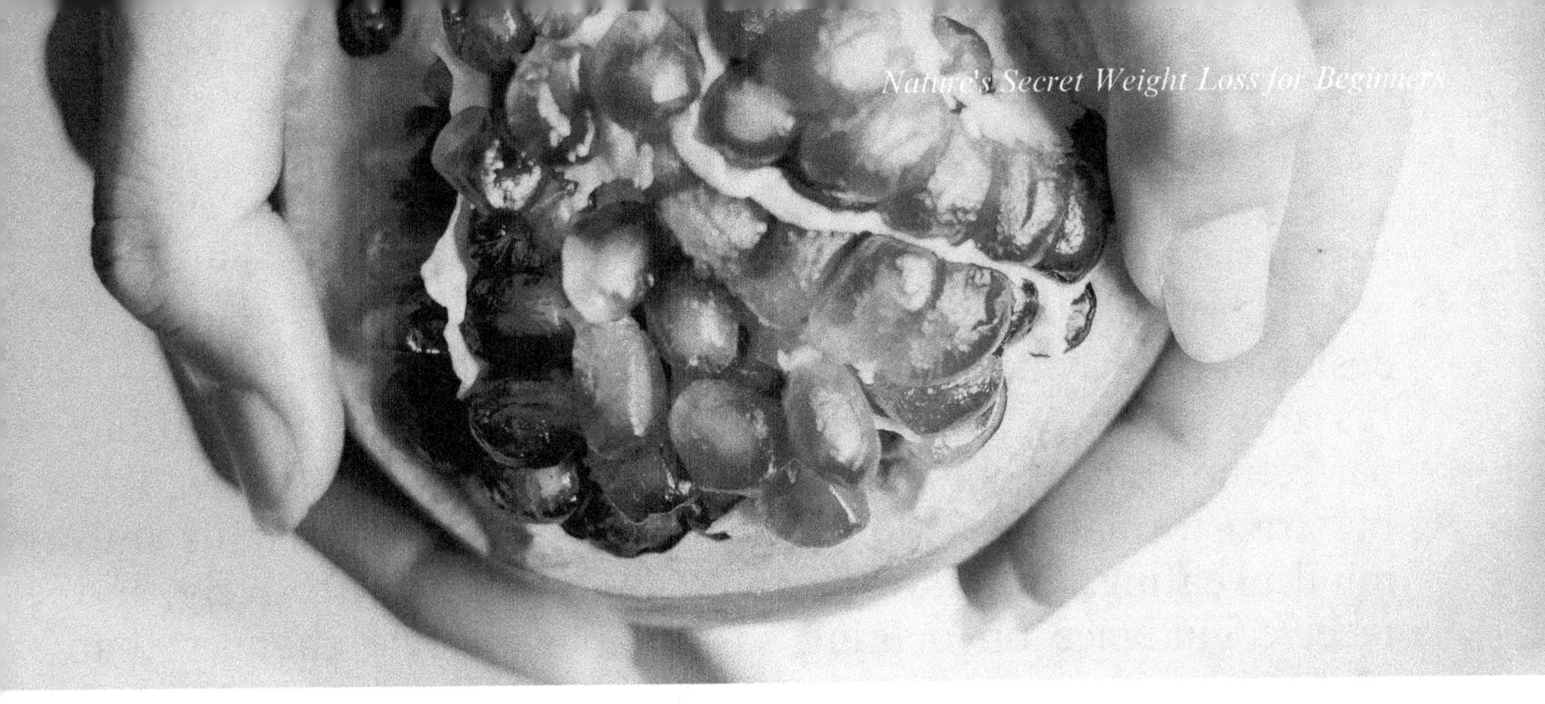

INTRODUCTION

Welcome to "Nature's Secret Weight Loss for Beginners . Congratulations on taking the first step towards a healthier, more vibrant you. In the fast-paced world we live in, it's easy to be drawn to quick fixes and trendy diets that promise instant results. However, true and lasting change comes from understanding and harnessing the power of nature's timeless wisdom.

In this book, we embark on a journey together to discover the natural, sustainable approaches that will not only help you shed excess weight but also nourish your body, mind, and soul. You'll learn how to embrace the abundance of fruits and vegetables, find alternatives to refined sugars, and develop habits that support your long-term health and wellness. We'll delve into the pitfalls of fad diets and explore why building healthy habits is the cornerstone of successful weight management.

From the importance of staying hydrated to the benefits of getting outside and connecting with nature, each chapter is designed to provide you with practical, actionable guidance.
It's important to remember that this journey is not about perfection, but about progress. Small, consistent steps lead to big transformations. Along the way, you'll gain insights into mindful eating, learn how to track your progress effectively, and receive guidance on making sustainable lifestyle changes that align with your unique needs and goals.

Through it all, remember that you are not alone. You have within you the power to unlock the secrets of natural, balanced living. Let this book be your guide and companion on your path to a healthier, happier you.
So, let's begin this journey together. Embrace the wisdom of nature, trust in your own inner strength, and let's uncover the secrets to a more vibrant, healthier you in 2023.

Warm regards,

[Janet R. Sheppard

The Importance of Natural Weight Loss Approaches

It is impossible to overestimate the significance of sustainable and natural weight loss techniques. In a society full of fad diets and fast fixes, it's crucial to realize the significant advantages of implementing a strategy based on the wisdom of nature.

Here are some basic Importance of Natural Weight Loss Approaches.

Long-Term Achievement: Gradual, consistent improvement is the main goal of natural weight loss approaches. Even though short remedies may result in a cycle of weight loss and gain, they can initially produce rapid benefits. Conversely, sustainable approaches emphasize the development of long-lasting routines and lifestyle modifications that are sustainable over time.

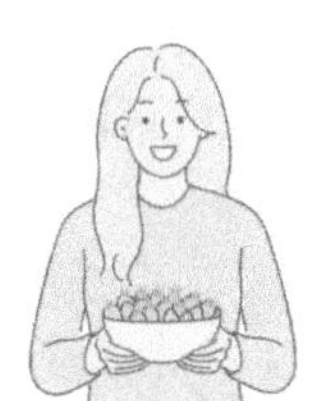

Nourishing the Body: Whole, nutrient-dense foods are the focus of natural methods of nourishing the body. In addition to aiding in weight loss, this also enhances general health and wellbeing.
It guarantees that you get the vital vitamins, minerals, and nourishment your body requires to work at its best.

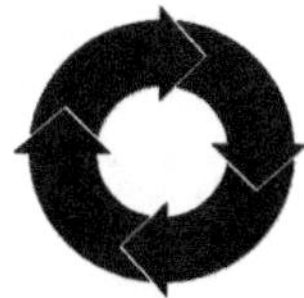 **Better Health Through Metabolic Process:** Techniques for losing weight that are sustainable also improve metabolic health. Making healthy eating and exercise a priority can help control insulin levels, lower inflammation, and improve metabolic efficiency. Consequently, this promotes sensible weight control.

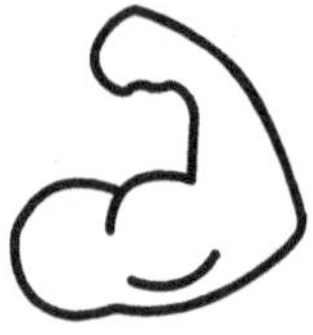 **Maintaining Muscle Mass**: Along with fat loss, crash diets and severe calorie restriction can cause muscle loss. The goal of natural approaches is to maintain lean muscle mass, which is essential for overall strength and vitality as well as a healthy metabolism.

Improved Mental Health: A healthy relationship with food and mindfulness are common components of natural weight loss techniques. This lowers the risk of developing disordered eating patterns or a negative body image by fostering a healthy mentality surrounding eating and self-image.

Diminished Chance of Nutritious Inadequacies: Nutrient deficiencies may result from rigid dietary habits or extreme diets. Natural approaches reduce the chance of lacking important nutrients by promoting a balanced diet rich in a range of foods.

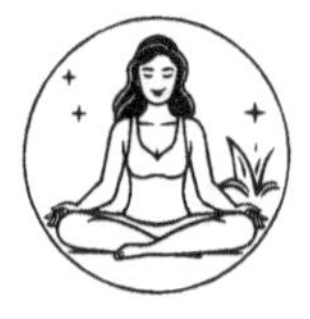 **Sustainable lifestyle change**: This can be achieved through natural weight loss approaches, which enable people to make long-lasting adjustments in their everyday routines. This is embracing an active lifestyle, finding joy in it, and implementing healthier diet and exercise routines.

How To Use This Book

1. **Read the Book Thoroughly:** Begin by reading the book from start to finish. This will give you a comprehensive overview of the natural and sustainable weight loss methods it advocates.

2. **Take Notes and Highlight Key Points**: As you read, take notes on important concepts, tips, and strategies that resonate with you. Highlight key points or passages that you find particularly insightful or actionable.

3. **Set Realistic Goals:** Based on the information in the book, set specific and achievable goals for your own weight loss journey. These goals should align with your personal needs, preferences, and circumstances.

4. **Implement the Recommendations:**
Start incorporating the recommended practices and strategies into your daily life. This could involve changes in your diet, exercise routine, sleep habits, and mindset.

5. **Experiment and Adapt:** Use the book as a guide, but be open to experimenting and finding what works best for you. Not every recommendation may fit your individual needs, so feel free to adapt the advice to suit your lifestyle.

6. **Tracking Your Progress**: Utilize the tracking tools and techniques provided in the book to monitor your progress. This could include keeping a food journal, recording your exercise routines, and noting changes in your weight and overall well-being

7. Stay Consistent: Consistency is key to seeing positive results. Stick to the natural and sustainable practices outlined in the book over time. Remember that gradual progress leads to lasting change.

8. Listen to Your Body: Pay attention to how your body responds to the changes you're making. Adjust your approach if needed based on your own feedback and intuition.

9. Seek Support and Accountability: If possible, find a support system or accountability partner. This could be a friend, family member, or an online community of individuals with similar goals.

10. Reflect and Reevaluate: Periodically reflect on your journey. Celebrate your achievements and identify areas where you may want to adjust your approach. Remember that it's a dynamic process.

11. Practice Patience and Self-Compassion: Understand that natural and sustainable weight loss takes time. Be patient with yourself and practice self-compassion, especially during moments of challenge or setbacks.

12. Incorporate Mindfulness and Enjoyment: Embrace the principles of mindful eating and exercise, and find joy in the process. Nourish your body and soul with practices that bring you fulfillment and satisfaction.

13. Share Your Journey: Consider sharing your experiences with others. Your insights and progress may inspire and support those around you who are also on a path to natural and sustainable weight loss

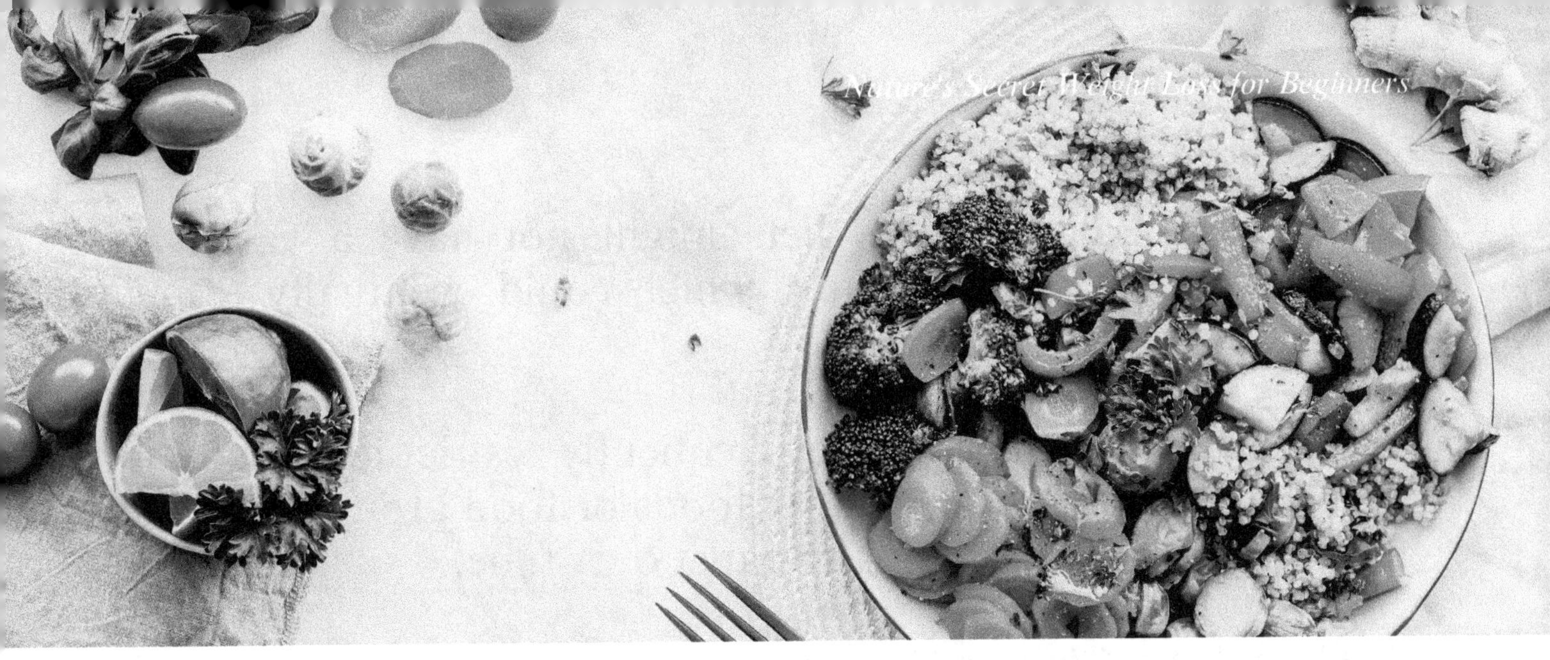

Pitfalls of Fad Diets

WHAT IS FAD DIETS?

Fad diets are rapid diets or weight reduction strategies that gain popularity due to media attention, celebrity endorsements, or word-of-mouth marketing. Usually, they guarantee quick weight loss by using extremely restricted or unusual dietary regimens. Fad diets, however, frequently lack scientific support and could not be long-term healthful or sustainable.

Fad diet characteristics could include:

1. Strong Restrictions: Fad diets frequently have strong limitations on the amount of calories consumed overall, on certain food groups, or on macronutrients (such as fats or carbs).

2. Quick Fix Mentality: Individuals looking for quick results may find their promises of quick, dramatic weight loss in a short amount of time appealing.

3. Lack of Balance: Fad diets might not have a varied and balanced dietary composition, which could eventually result in nutritional deficiencies.

4. Limited Food Choices: They frequently restrict dietary options to a small number of particular foods or food groups, which can make it challenging to stick to a diet over time.

5. Unrealistic Claims: Fad diets often make exaggerated claims about their effectiveness without substantial scientific evidence to support them.

6. Elimination of Entire Food Groups: Some fad diets completely eliminate certain food groups, which can lead to potential nutrient imbalances and deficiencies.

Understanding the Drawbacks And Consequences of Fad Diets

Understanding the drawbacks of fad diets is crucial for making informed decisions about weight loss strategies. Here are some key considerations:

1. Unsustainability:

Issue: Fad diets often involve extreme restrictions or drastic changes in eating patterns that are difficult to maintain over the long term.

Consequence: While they may lead to initial weight loss, the strict nature of fad diets can be hard to sustain. This often results in individuals reverting back to their previous eating habits, leading to regained weight.

2. Nutritional Deficiencies:

Issue: Fad diets may eliminate entire food groups or severely limit nutrient intake, potentially leading to deficiencies in essential vitamins, minerals, and macronutrients.

Consequence: Prolonged deficiency can have negative effects on overall health, potentially causing fatigue, weakened immune function, and other health issues.

3. Metabolic Adaptation:

Issue: Rapid weight loss from fad diets can lead to a reduction in metabolic rate. The body may adapt to lower calorie intake by slowing down metabolism.

Consequence: This can make it harder to continue losing weight and easier to regain lost weight when normal eating patterns are resumed.

4. Muscle Loss:

Issue: Some fad diets can lead to loss of lean muscle mass along with fat. This is especially common in very low-calorie diets.

Consequence: Muscle loss can lead to a lower metabolic rate and decreased strength and physical function.

5. Negative Impact on Mental Health:

Issue: The extreme nature of fad diets can lead to feelings of deprivation, frustration, and even guilt around food choices.

Consequence: This can contribute to an unhealthy relationship with food and body image, potentially leading to disordered eating patterns or negative self-perception.

6. Potential Health Risks:

Issue: Some fad diets may not provide all the essential nutrients needed for optimal health, potentially leading to health complications.

Consequence: Depending on the specific diet, risks can range from nutrient deficiencies to more serious health issues like heart problems or electrolyte imbalances.

7. Lack of Individualization:

Issue: Fad diets are typically designed for a broad audience and may not take into account an individual's unique nutritional needs, preferences, or underlying health conditions.

Consequence: What works for one person may not work for another, and following a one-size-fits-all approach may not lead to optimal results.

Why Sustainable Approaches Are Key

Sustainable approaches to weight loss are considered the key for several important reasons:

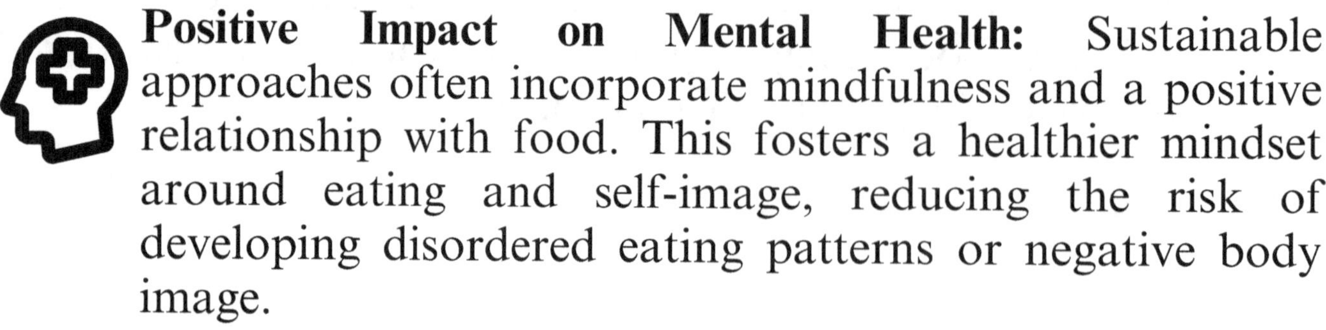

Reduces Risk of Weight Cycling: Sustainable approaches help minimize the likelihood of weight cycling, which is the repeated loss and regain of weight. This pattern can be detrimental to both physical and mental health.

Positive Impact on Mental Health: Sustainable approaches often incorporate mindfulness and a positive relationship with food. This fosters a healthier mindset around eating and self-image, reducing the risk of developing disordered eating patterns or negative body image.

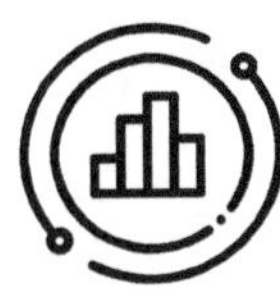 **Flexible and Adaptable:** Sustainable methods are flexible and adaptable to individual preferences, making them easier to integrate into your lifestyle. This increases the likelihood of long-term adherence.

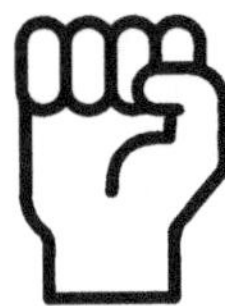 **Empowerment and Self-Confidence:** Achieving weight loss through sustainable methods fosters a sense of empowerment and self-confidence. Knowing that you have the tools and knowledge to take control of your health is a powerful motivator.

 **Lifestyle Integration:** Sustainable approaches are designed to be integrated into your daily life seamlessly. They encourage a balanced approach to nutrition, exercise, sleep, and overall well-being.

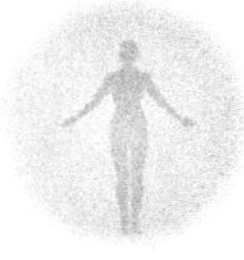 **Less Likely to Cause Health Complications:** Sustainable methods are generally less likely to lead to health complications compared to extreme or fad diets. They provide a safer and more balanced approach to achieving and maintaining a healthy weight.

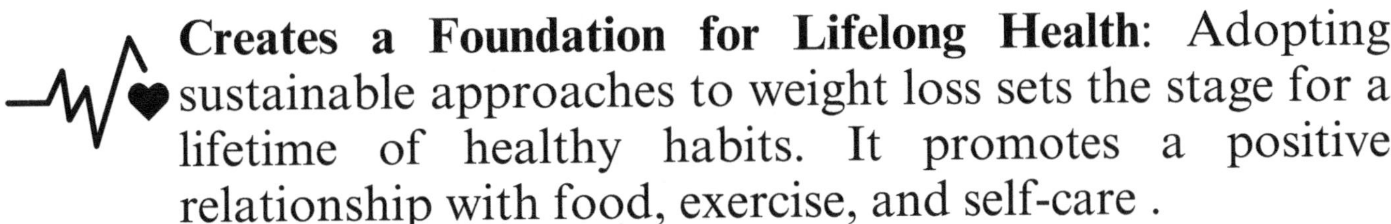 **Creates a Foundation for Lifelong Health:** Adopting sustainable approaches to weight loss sets the stage for a lifetime of healthy habits. It promotes a positive relationship with food, exercise, and self-care .

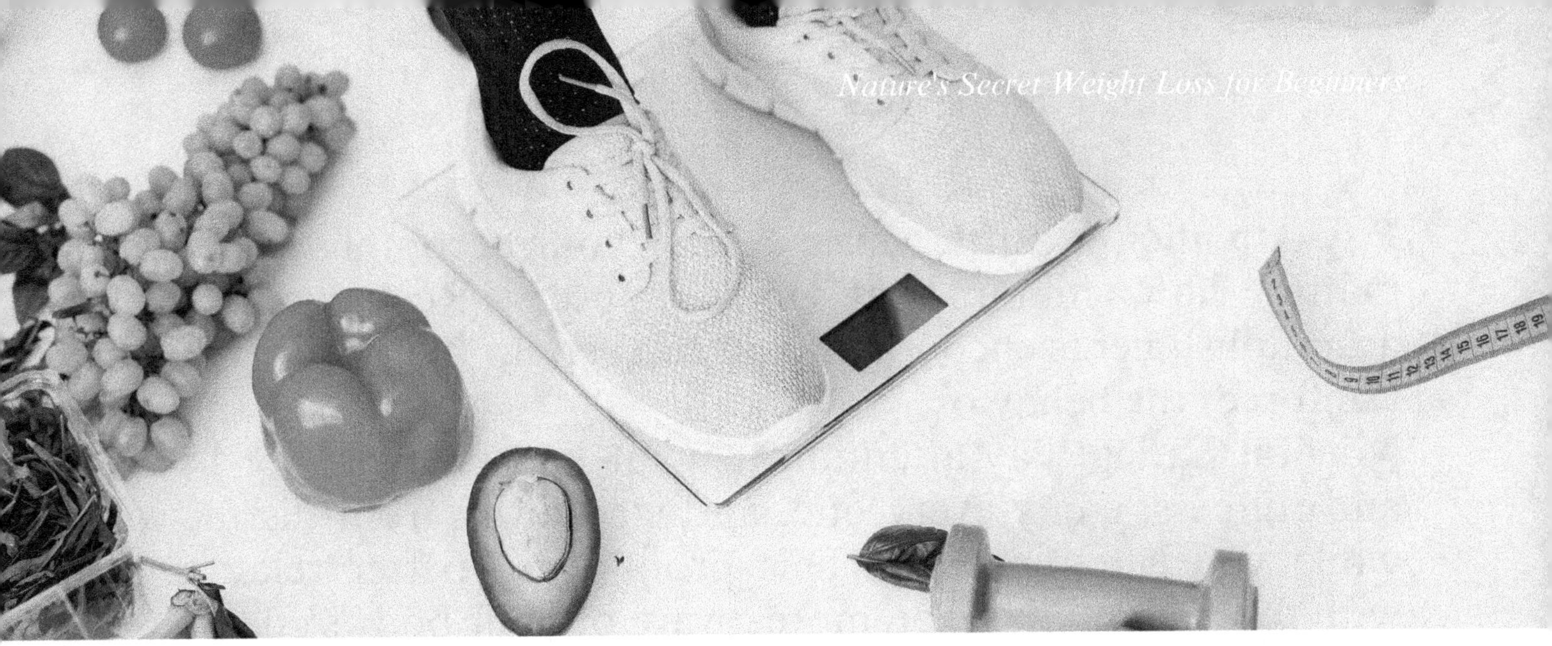

Building Weight Loss Habits

Starting a weight reduction journey is about developing long-lasting, health-promoting behaviors that will benefit you in the long run, not simply about losing weight. Developing these habits is essential to reaching and keeping a healthy weight over time. The following are some crucial ideas to think about:

Initiate Small and Expand Gradually: Start by concentrating on one or two specific habits at a time. After those get deeply inbuilt, you can add more. This strategy raises the possibility of success while reducing overwhelm.

Set Specific, Achievable Goals: Establish goals that are in line with your overall weight loss aims. Having specific goals gives you direction, whether it's eating more veggies or making time for regular exercise.

Establish a Schedule: Routines aid in the formation of new habits. Your brain becomes programmed to identify a behaviour with a specific moment or situation when you execute it consistently at the same time or in the same context.

Pay Attention to Little Wins: Honor your accomplishments, no matter how minor they may appear. Recognizing your accomplishments encourages you to keep up the good work and reinforces the behavior.

Mindful Eating: Pay attention to your body's signals of hunger and fullness, enjoy every bite, and stay away from distractions while you eat mindfully. This promotes a better relationship with food and makes you more aware of your body's cues.

Install Positive Habits in Place of Negative Ones: Determine which behaviors are impeding your growth and try to replace them with more healthful ones. For instance, to combat sedentary behaviors, replace sugary snacks with full fruits or include a daily stroll.

Accountability and Support: Share your goals with someone you trust, such as a friend, family member, or support group. Having someone to share your progress with can provide encouragement and motivation.

Learn from Setbacks: It's normal to face challenges and setbacks along the way. Instead of viewing them as failures, see them as learning opportunities. Analyze what went wrong and use that knowledge to adjust your approach.

Incorporate Variety: Incorporating a variety of foods and exercises into your routine keeps things interesting and prevents boredom. This also ensures you receive a wide range of nutrients for optimal health.

Practice Self-Compassion: Be kind and understanding with yourself. Recognize that building new habits is a journey, and it's okay to have moments of struggle. Treat yourself with the same kindness and encouragement you would offer to a friend.

The Power of Habits in Achieving Lasting Weight Loss

Habits are the unseen forces that mold our everyday existence, affecting our decisions, actions, and, in the end, our results. Utilizing the power of habits is one of the best methods for attaining long-term weight reduction. This is the reason why:

Automated Selection of Actions: Habits avoid the requirement for continuous deliberate decision-making. When a behavior develops into a habit, it becomes an instinctive, natural reaction to a certain stimulus or circumstance. This lessens the mental effort needed to continuously make wise decisions.

Deciding to Reduce Decision Fatigue: Throughout the day, making a lot of decisions can cause decision fatigue, which makes it more difficult to keep your composure and self-control. By automating some acts, habits reduce this load and free up mental energy for other activities.

Triggers and Cues: A lot of the time, certain signs or circumstances set off a habit. By being aware of these indicators, you may intentionally create an environment that encourages healthy behaviors. To promote better snacking habits, for instance, arrange fruits and vegetables in the refrigerator at eye level.

Building Stronger Positive Feedback Loops: A positive feedback loop is created when positive habits produce beneficial results.

Your incentive to maintain healthy habits is strengthened when you reap the rewards of such actions, such as better mood or more energy.

Overcoming Opposition: Adopting a new behavior can be difficult since it frequently calls for motivation and deliberate effort. On the other hand, a behavior that becomes ingrained becomes easier and needs less conscious effort, which makes it more long-term sustainable.

Shaping Identity: Our sense of self is entwined with our habits. A healthy action becomes a part of who you are when you make it a habit. For instance, reinforcing healthy eating habits or an enjoyment of exercise are examples of self-reinforcement activities.

Switching to Change: Routines are flexible. Habits can be adjusted to fit new routines or settings when circumstances change. You can continue to practice healthy habits even when faced with obstacles in life thanks to this adaptability.

Building Momentum: Adopting further healthy habits can be facilitated by the establishment of a positive habit that sets off a cascade effect. For instance, consistent exercise may enhance sleep, which in turn encourages healthier eating decisions.

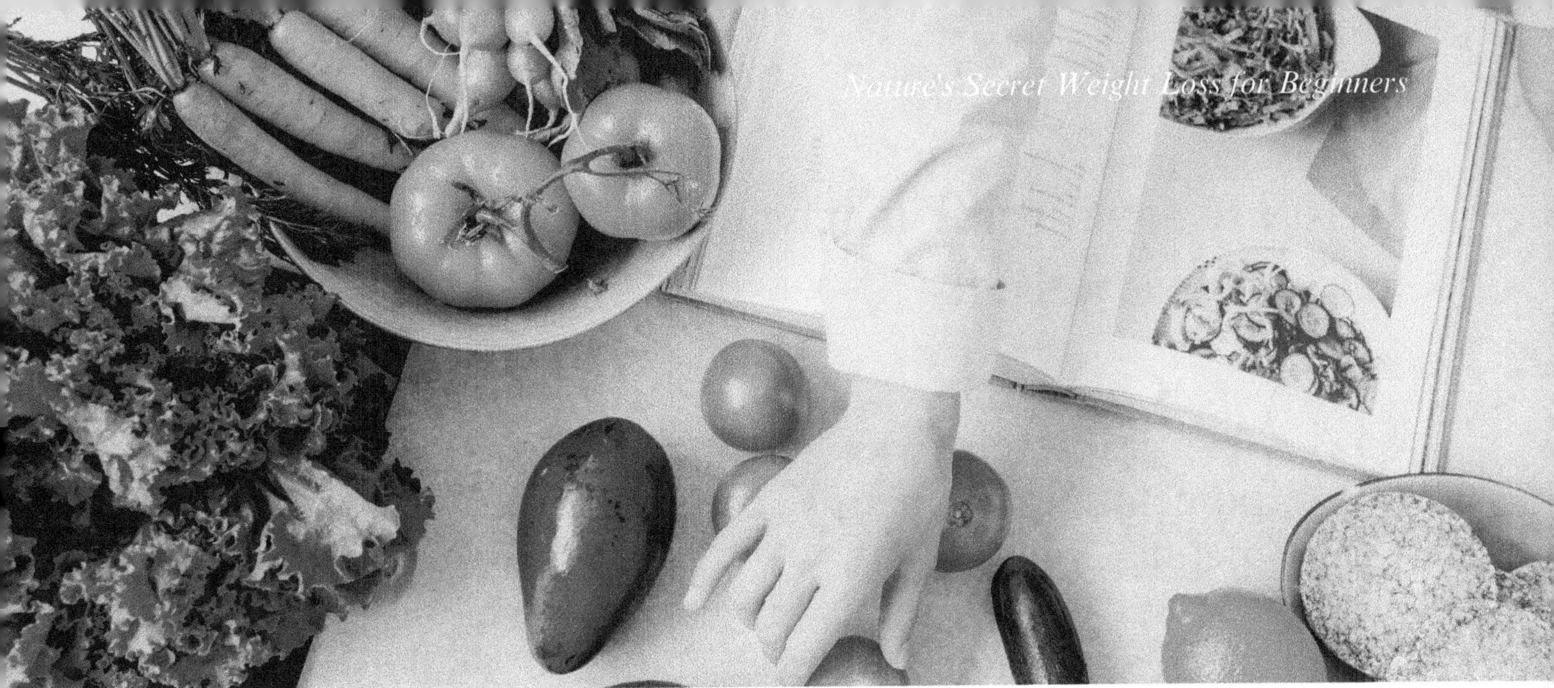

EATING MORE FRUITS AND VEGETABLES

The basis of a nutritious, well-balanced diet is an increased intake of fruits and vegetables. They are abundant in fiber, antioxidants, and other nutrients that support general health.

Many fruits are high in fiber and low in calories, which may help with weight loss. Certain fruits, such as melons, berries, and apples, might also make you feel more full.

Fruit is a natural snack that is high in fiber, vitamins, and other nutrients that help maintain a balanced diet.

Fruit may aid in weight loss because it is often high in fiber and low in calories.

Consuming fruit is associated with a reduced body weight as well as a decreased risk of heart disease, diabetes, high blood pressure, and cancer.

Here are some fruits that you may include in your diet to help you lose weight:

Citrus fruits

The grapefruit, which is a hybrid of an orange and a pomelo, is frequently connected to weight loss and dieting.

Measuring 123 grams (g), half a grapefruit offers 51% of the Daily Value (DV) of vitamin C while only offering 37 calories. A tiny quantity of vitamin A is also present in red variants.

Additionally, grapefruit releases sugar into the circulatory system more slowly due to its low glycemic index (GI). The evidence for a low-GI diet's ability to help with weight loss and maintenance is weak.

Furthermore, naringenin, a flavonoid with anti-inflammatory and antioxidant qualities that may guard against diabetes and heart disease, is abundant in grapefruit.

Grapefruit is high in vitamin C and low in calories. It could be a nutritious snack before main meals to help you eat less overall.

Apples

Apples are high in fiber and low in calories, with 116 calories and 5.4 g of fiber per large apple (223g).

They have also been shown to aid with weight loss.

According to a review of research, apples contain polyphenols that may help reduce visceral fat buildup in people with varying BMI and weights.

According to research, apple peels contain antioxidants and helpful chemicals that may lower the incidence of obesity.

According to research, apples are best consumed whole rather than juiced to lessen hunger and appetite.

Apple polyphenol extract, which is derived from one of the fruit's natural constituents, has also been associated to higher HDL (good) cholesterol levels and lower inflammation.

Apples are low in calories, high in fiber, and very filling. Studies indicate that they may support weight loss.

3. **Berries**

Berries are nutritious powerhouses with few calories.

For instance, just 64 calories and 36% of the Daily Value (DV) for vitamin C, manganese, and 12% for vitamin K may be found in one cup (123 g) of raspberries.

Strawberries include less than 50 calories per cup (152 g), 3 g of dietary fiber, 99% of the daily value for vitamin C, and 26% of the DV for manganese.

Berries filling as well.

Berries may also help lower blood pressure, cholesterol, and inflammation, all of which may be especially beneficial for those who are overweight.

Berries are rich in essential vitamins and low in calories. They might also be beneficial for blood pressure, inflammation, and cholesterol..

Advice for increasing daily fruit and vegetable intake:

1. Fruit should be kept visible.To stimulate a sweet tooth, pile a dish full of ready-to-eat, thoroughly cleaned fruits or put chopped, vibrant fruits in a glass bowl and refrigerate.

2. Examine the produce section and choose something else. A balanced diet is all about color and variety. Try to include one serving of each of the following foods on most days: citrus fruits, legumes (beans and peas), red and yellow or orange fruits and vegetables, dark green leafy vegetables, and red fruits and vegetables. Let the potatoes go.

3. Select a variety of veggies that are high in nutrients and have exceptionally slow digesting carbs. Make it a meal now. Attempt preparing something fresh that include more vegetables.

The Nutritional Benefits of a Plant-Forward Diet

A plant-forward diet places a strong emphasis on whole, minimally processed plant-based foods, such as fruits, vegetables, whole grains, legumes, nuts, and seeds. Here are some of the significant nutritional benefits associated with incorporating more fruits and vegetables into your diet:

Abundance of Vitamins and Minerals: Fruits and vegetables are rich sources of essential vitamins and minerals like vitamin C, potassium, folate, and various phytonutrients. These nutrients are crucial for supporting overall health, immune function, and vitality.

Dietary Fiber for Digestive Health: They are high in dietary fiber, which aids in digestion, regulates blood sugar levels, and promotes a feeling of fullness, helping to manage appetite and prevent overeating.

Antioxidants for Cellular Health: Fruits and vegetables are packed with antioxidants like vitamins A, C, and E, as well as various phytochemicals. These compounds help protect cells from oxidative damage, which can contribute to chronic diseases and aging.

Lower Caloric Density: Most fruits and vegetables are low in calories but high in volume and nutrient density. This means you can eat larger portions without consuming excess calories, which supports weight management.

Heart-Healthy Nutrients: Many fruits and vegetables are rich in nutrients like potassium, which helps regulate blood pressure, and fiber, which contributes to heart health by managing cholesterol levels.

Reduced Risk of Chronic Diseases: A diet high in fruits and vegetables has been associated with a lower risk of chronic diseases such as heart disease, certain cancers, and type 2 diabetes.

Weight Management: The fiber content in fruits and vegetables helps promote a feeling of fullness, which can help control appetite and prevent overeating.

Improved Skin Health: The vitamins and antioxidants in fruits and vegetables, such as vitamin C and beta-carotene, contribute to healthy, radiant skin by promoting collagen production and protecting against UV damage.

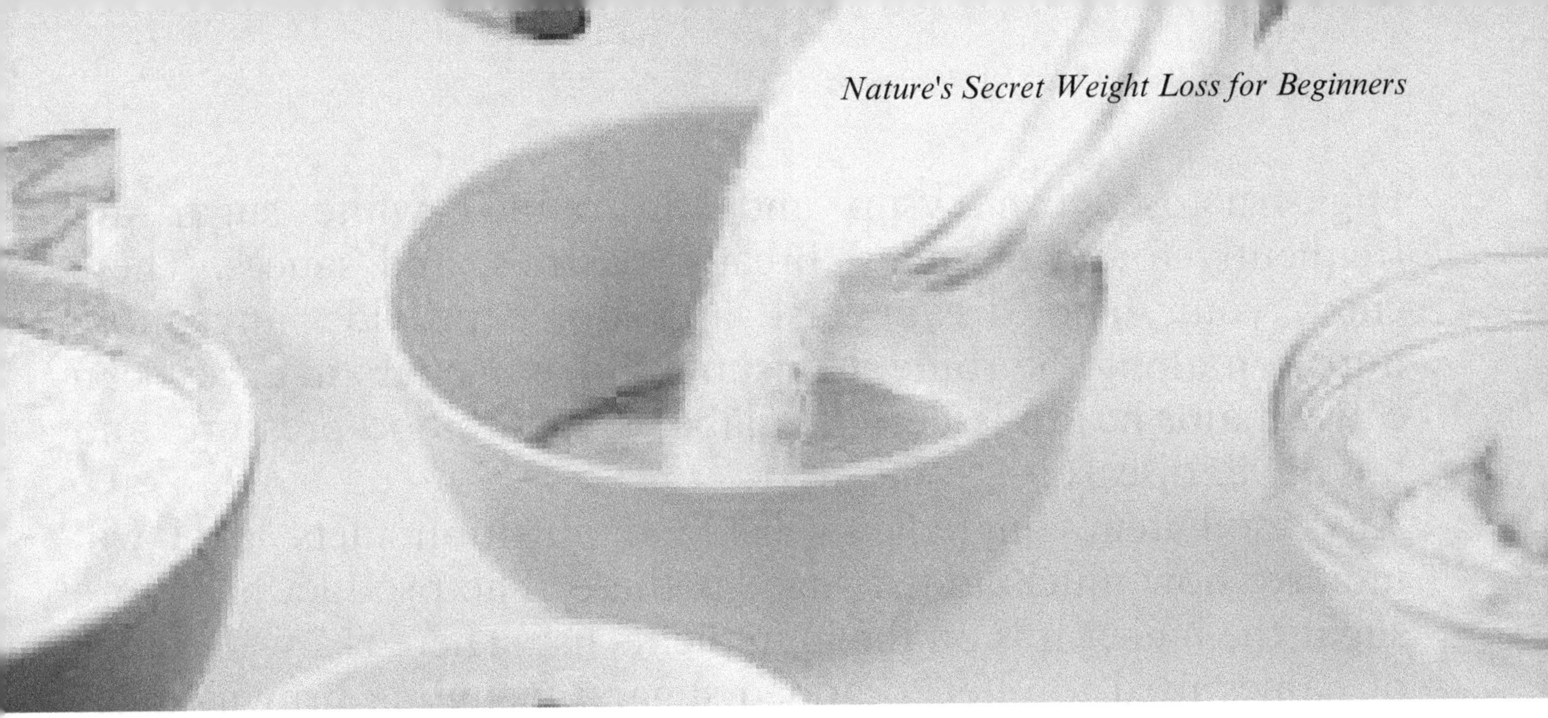

Seeking Alternative Sugars

What are alternatives to sugar?

Let me make it clear that sugar isn't intrinsically unhealthy before discussing sugar substitutes. It's actually essential to your wellness. Your body uses glucose, a type of sugar that is produced when carbs are broken down, as your main energy source to keep your body and brain operating. Contrary to what several popular diet fads claim, you may suffer from health issues and symptoms including poor energy, difficulty sleeping, and mental fog if you don't consume enough carbohydrates and sugars.

Consuming the appropriate types of sugar rather than avoiding it should be the main objective. The added sugars that are processed and refined to provide extreme sweetness without much content make up a large portion of the diet of the modern American.

High-fructose corn syrup and ultrarefined white sugar are frequently found in sodas, breads, pastries, and sauces. These enter your bloodstream fast and don't provide any more nutrition along the route. Consuming these sugars in excess can cause major health issues like diabetes, high blood pressure, and fatty liver disease.

Any food item's ingredients list and nutrition facts label will indicate how much added sugar is there. The product has more sugar the higher it is on the ingredients list. There is a wide range of names used to refer to added sugars, including brown sugar, corn syrup, dextrose, fructose, glucose, high-fructose corn syrup, malt syrup, maltose, and sucrose.

Natural sugars, on the other hand, are present in many foods naturally and are either unprocessed or just minimally processed. For instance, fruits provide a lot of fiber in addition to fructose, giving your body a well-balanced mix of nutrients. In addition to being naturally sweet, honey and maple syrup are also high in vitamins, minerals, and antioxidants.

Exploring Natural Sweeteners and Sugar Substitutes

While moderate consumption of typical refined sugars can contribute to a balanced diet, many individuals are looking for alternatives for a variety of reasons, such as controlling blood sugar levels, cutting calories, or just trying out new flavors. The following are some popular natural sugar alternatives and sweeteners:

1. **Honey**: Honey has a deep flavor and is a natural sweetener. It has long been valued for its nutritional content in addition to its inherent sweetness. Honey has a variety of healthy plant components and antioxidants since bees make it from plant nectar during pollination. It should still be used sparingly though, as it is still a kind of added sugar.

2. **Maple Syrup:** Maple syrup, another well-liked natural sweetener, has taken the place of honey on a lot of pancakes. Pancakes should be avoided if you're trying to cut back on sugar, but you should save the syrup, which is made from maple tree sap. In comparison to refined sugars, it is a little more nutrient-dense since it includes certain minerals and antioxidants.

3. **Stevia**: The leaves of the stevia plant are used to make this calorie-free, naturally occurring sweetener. Because it's considerably sweeter than sugar, you only need a small amount. It's a well-liked option for people trying to cut back on sugar and calories.
Stevia is a non-nutritive sugar replacement that has very little calories. It's sweetening without adding much more, which can be exactly what you're seeking for while reducing your sugar intake. Stevia has also been linked to lower cholesterol and blood sugar levels. Remember that a lot of stevia products on the market include sugar alcohols or other processed chemicals, so be sure to do your homework before using them.

4. **Monk Fruit Extract**: Made from the monk fruit, monk fruit extract is a naturally occurring sweetener. It has no calories and no carbs, but it's really sweet. It's a good choice for people looking for a low-calorie substitute.

5. **Coconut Sugar:** The sap of coconut palm plants is used to make coconut sugar. It may have less of an effect on blood sugar levels because it has a lower glycemic index than ordinary sugar.

6. **Date Paste**: Dates and water are blended to make date paste. It's a nutrient- and fiber-rich natural sweetener. It works well in a variety of recipes as a whole-food sweetener.

7. **blended fruit**: Raw fruits are hard to beat for a more nutritionally balanced sugar substitute. Fruit juice and sugar additions can cause blood sugar spikes, however the dietary fiber in raw fruits helps with digestion and slows down sugar metabolism. Consuming meals high in fiber can also help you consume fewer calories overall and minimize your chance of developing heart disease.

Fruits that have been pureed offer many of the same advantages and can be used as sweeteners in other dishes. Many recipes can be made with applesauce in place of eggs.

How to Reduce Added Sugars in Your Diet

Reducing added sugars in your diet can have significant health benefits, including improved blood sugar control, weight management, and reduced risk of chronic diseases. Here are some practical tips to help you cut down on added sugars:

Read Labels: Check food labels for added sugars. They can hide under various names like sucrose, glucose, fructose, high-fructose corn syrup, and more.

Limit Sugary Beverages: Avoid or reduce consumption of sugary drinks like sodas, fruit juices, and sweetened teas. Opt for water, herbal teas, or naturally flavored water instead.

Choose Whole Fruits: me Instead of reaching for sugary snacks or desserts, opt for whole fruits which provide natural sweetness along with fiber and nutrients.

Opt for Unsweetened Options: Choose unsweetened versions of products like yogurt, oatmeal, and nut milk. You can add natural sweeteners like fruits or a small amount of honey or maple syrup if needed.

Cook at Home: When you prepare meals at home, you have control over the ingredients. You can use natural sweeteners or reduce sugar content in recipes.

Be Mindful of Condiments: Some condiments, like ketchup and salad dressings, can contain hidden sugars. Look for options with no added sugars or make your own at home.

Gradually Reduce Sugar in Recipes: When baking or cooking, try gradually reducing the amount of sugar used in recipes. Your taste buds will adjust over time.

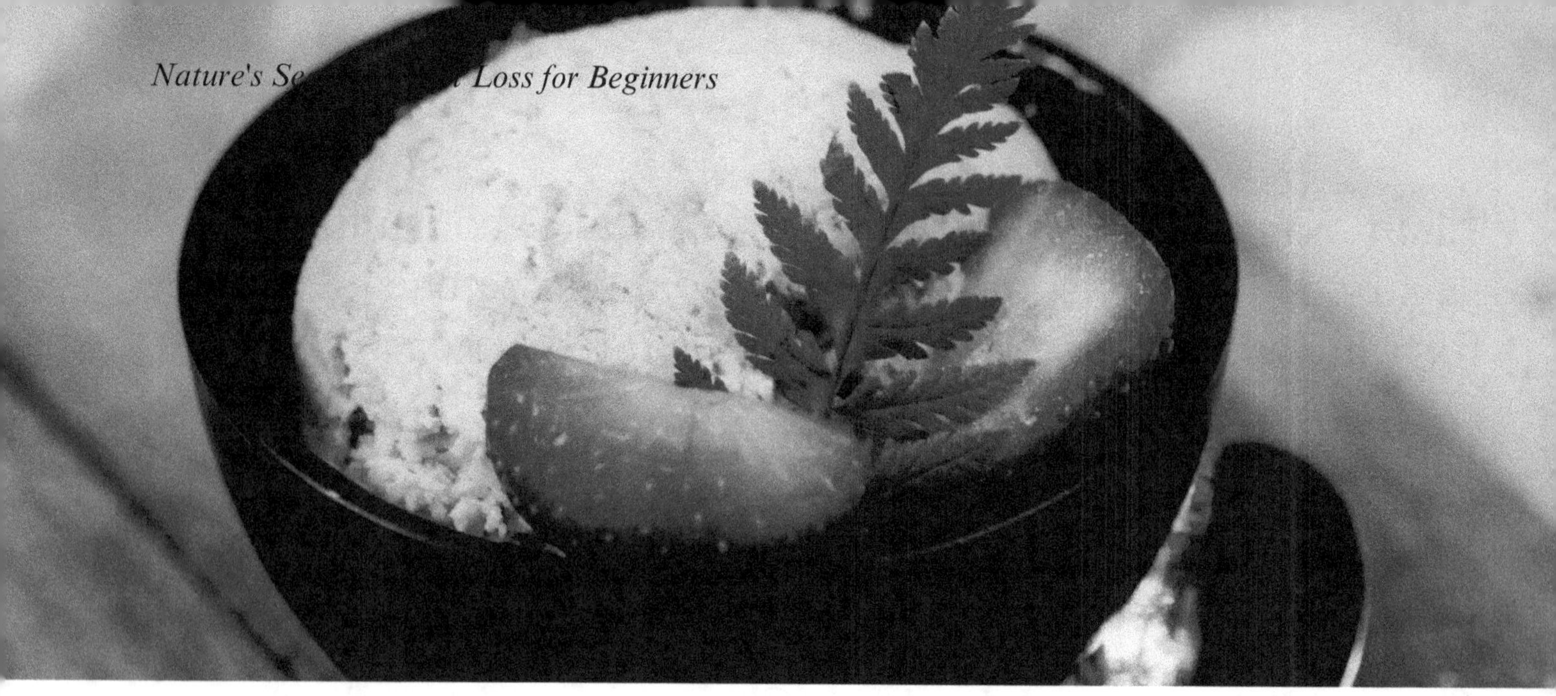

Sweetening Foods in a Healthier Way

If you're looking to sweeten foods and beverages in a healthier way, consider these alternatives:

Fruits: Fresh or dried fruits like bananas, dates, and figs can be blended or mashed and used to naturally sweeten dishes.

Cinnamon and Nutmeg: These spices can add warmth and a hint of sweetness to foods and beverages without the need for additional sugars.

Vanilla Extract: A small amount of pure vanilla extract can enhance the natural sweetness of foods without adding extra sugar.

Herbal Teas: Naturally sweet herbal teas like chamomile or mint can be a flavorful, low-calorie alternative to sugary beverages

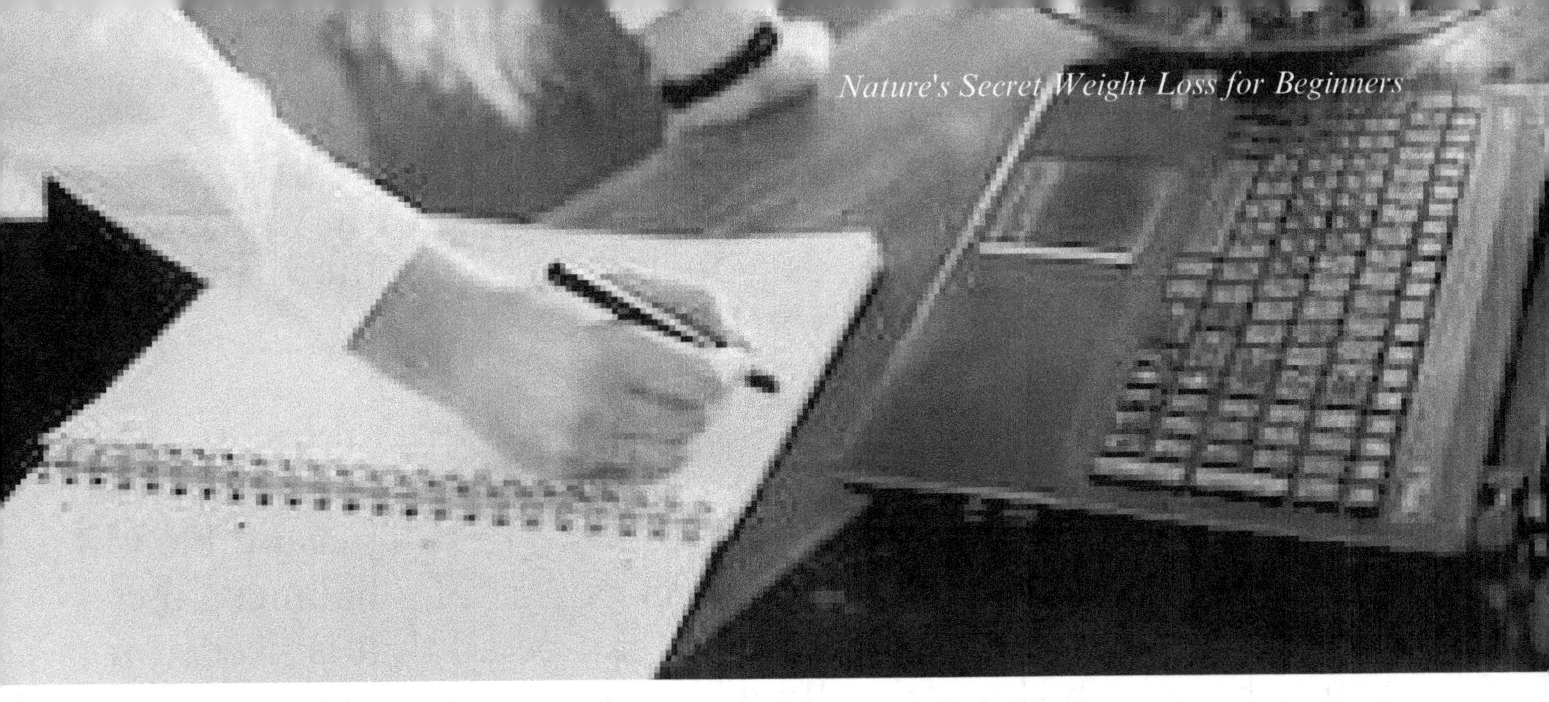

PLANNING MORE MEALS

Organizing your meals more thoroughly will help you reach and stay within a healthy body weight range, better control the quality of your food, and manage your nutrition. It entails planning and preparing meals in advance, which has various advantages for your general health.

This may surprise you, but there is no specific diet that you must adhere to in order to lose weight.

It's not always required to follow certain dietary regimens, like low-carb or vegan diets, to lose weight in a healthy, long-term fashion. However, research has shown that certain diets can help people lose weight.

Meal preparation is an excellent tool since it allows you to enjoy a nutrient-dense meal that suits your unique preferences and needs rather than adhering to a rigid, set schedule. When time is of the essence, the planning component enables you to prepare healthy meals.

since nothing is totally "off-limits," you have greater opportunity to choose foods you like and are more likely to enjoy the meals and snacks you consume.

In light of this, certain meals, like fruits and vegetables, are very nutrient-dense and have been associated with weight loss, while other items, like pastries and doughnuts, are still acceptable but ought to be consumed in moderation as part of a balanced diet. A well-rounded, nutrient-dense diet can be all that is needed for a healthy, weight-loss-friendly diet. Making ensuring you're in a calorie deficit, which encourages fat loss, is the most crucial component of weight loss.

This does not, however, imply that you must follow a rigid low-calorie diet. Alternatively, consider reducing your intake of some high-calorie, low-nutrient refined foods, selecting nutrient-dense, full foods more frequently, and increasing your regular physical exercise.
This will enable you to reduce your caloric intake while maintaining a sense of fullness and nourishment.

Importance of Meal Planning in Weight Management

Meal planning is a crucial component of successful weight management. It involves preparing and organizing meals ahead of time, which offers several benefits:

Portion Control: By planning meals in advance, you can portion out appropriate serving sizes, helping to prevent overeating and maintain a balanced calorie intake.

Nutrient-Dense Choices: Meal planning allows you to choose a variety of nutrient-dense foods, including fruits, vegetables, lean proteins, and whole grains, which support overall health and weight loss.

Reduced Impulse Eating: When meals are planned, you're less likely to grab unhealthy, convenience foods on the go. This helps you make more mindful and nutritious food choices.

Time and Money Savings: Planning meals in advance can save time and money by reducing the need for last-minute takeout or impromptu trips to the grocery store.

Stress Reduction: Knowing what you'll be eating ahead of time can reduce decision fatigue and alleviate stress associated with mealtime.

Balanced Nutrition: Meal planning enables you to ensure that your meals are balanced, providing a mix of macronutrients (carbohydrates, protein, and fats) and micronutrients (vitamins and minerals) necessary for sustained energy and overall well-being.

Practical Tips for Effective Meal Preparation

Here are some practical tips for effective meal preparation:

1. Set Aside Specific Time for Planning: Dedicate a specific time each week to plan your meals. This could be a weekend afternoon or any other convenient time for you.

2. **Choose Balanced Recipes:** Opt for recipes that include a mix of lean proteins, whole grains, plenty of vegetables, and healthy fats. This ensures you're getting a wide range of nutrients.

3. **Batch Cooking**: Prepare larger quantities of certain dishes that can be stored and eaten over multiple days. This saves time and ensures you have healthy options readily available.

4. **Use Storage Containers**: Invest in a variety of reusable containers in different sizes to store and portion out meals. This makes it easier to grab a balanced meal when you're on the go.

5. **Plan for Snacks**: Include healthy snacks like fruits, nuts, and yogurt in your meal plan to prevent reaching for less nutritious options when you're hungry between meals.

6. **Consider Dietary Preferences and Restrictions**: Take into account any dietary preferences, allergies, or restrictions when planning meals. This ensures that your meals align with your specific needs and goals.

Balancing Nutrients for Sustained Energy and Weight Loss

Balancing nutrients in your meals is crucial for sustained energy levels and supporting weight loss efforts. Here are some key principles to keep in mind:

Incorporate Lean Proteins: Include lean protein sources like poultry, fish, beans, tofu, and legumes in your meals. Protein helps with satiety and supports muscle maintenance.

Choose Complex Carbohydrates: Opt for whole grains like brown rice, quinoa, whole wheat bread, and oats. These provide a steady release of energy and help stabilize blood sugar levels.

Prioritize Healthy Fats: Include sources of healthy fats such as avocados, nuts, seeds, olive oil, and fatty fish like salmon. These fats provide essential nutrients and contribute to a feeling of fullness.

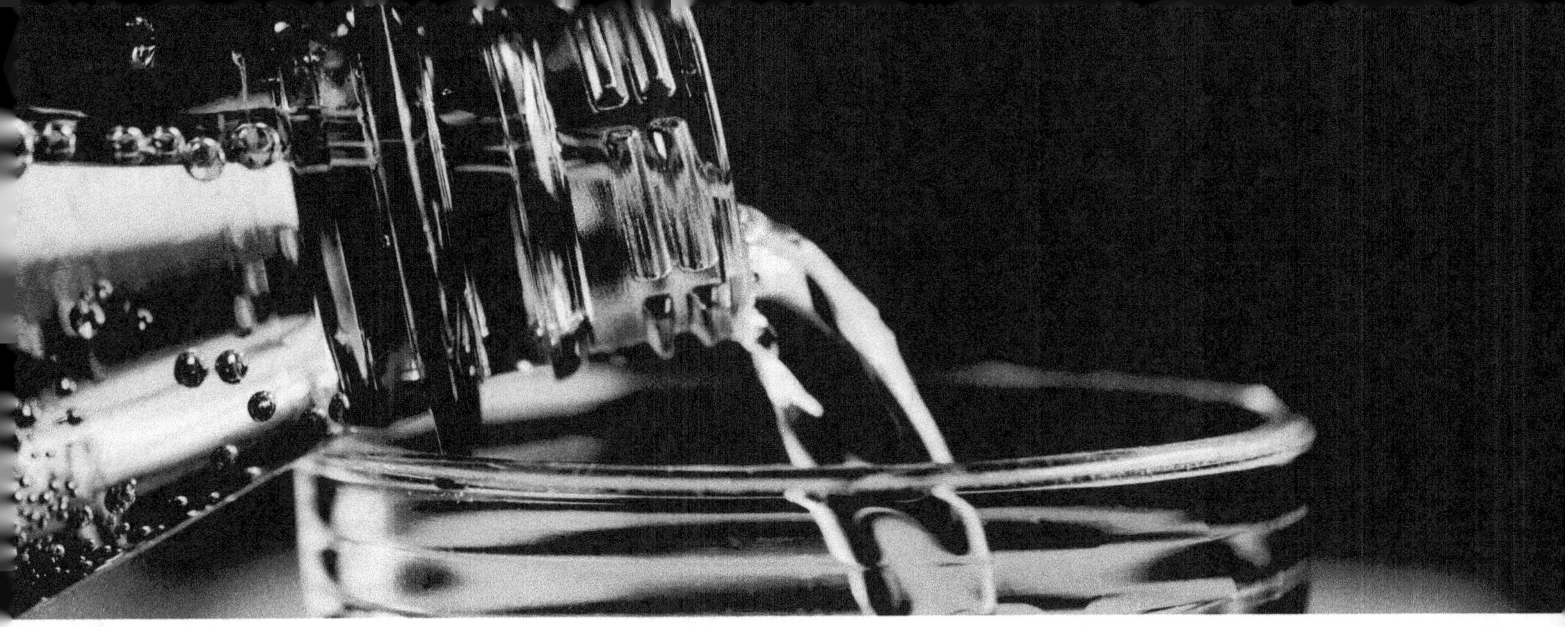

Drinking Water / Hydration

Maintaining general health and wellbeing, which are linked to weight loss, requires adequate hydration. Your body cannot operate as well when dehydrated, which can result in weight gain.

Drinking enough water is essential for managing weight in general. You're more likely to make good decisions, like eating well and getting regular exercise, when you're properly hydrated.
In order to lose weight, how much water should you drink?

Adult men should drink 15.5 cups (3.7 liters) of fluid per day, whereas adult women should drink 11.5 cups (2.7 liters) per day, according to the National Academies of Sciences, Engineering, and Medicine. But if you're attempting to lose weight, live in a hot climate, or are physically active, you might need to drink extra water.
If you're unsure how much water you need, start with eight glasses each day and observe how you feel. You can increase or decrease your consumption as needed.

The Role of Hydration in Weight Loss and Overall Health

In addition to being crucial for preserving general health, hydration is important for weight loss. The following are some essential details on how crucial it is to stay hydrated:

Control of Body Functions: Water is essential for controlling body temperature, digestion, circulation, and waste removal, among other processes. Sufficient hydration facilitates these processes' effective performance.

Appetite Regulation: Maintaining enough hydration levels might assist with appetite control. Sometimes, people confuse their thirst for hunger, which results in overindulging in calories. Water consumption can aid in distinguishing between the two feelings.

Metabolism and Calorie Burning: A healthy metabolism is supported by enough water. According to studies, consuming adequate water can momentarily increase metabolism, facilitating the burning of calories.

Optimal activity Performance: Hydration is essential for optimal performance during activity. Dehydration can impair one's strength, endurance, and general athletic performance.

Improved Cognitive Function: Sustaining cognitive function requires enough hydration. Reduced concentration, alertness, and mental clarity can result from even minor dehydration.

Detoxification and Waste Removal: Urine from water helps the body eliminate waste materials and pollutants. Kidney function and general detoxification both benefit from this.

Strategies for Staying Hydrated Throughout the Day

Keeping enough water in your body is a daily task. The following are some tips to keep you hydrated:

Set Reminders: Remind yourself to drink water at regular times throughout the day by setting alarms, using apps, or writing down physical reminders.

Bring a Water Bottle: Develop the practice of routinely sipping from a reusable water bottle that you always carry with you. This is a visual cue to drink plenty of water.

Monitor Urine Color: Observe the hue of your pee. Light-colored, pale pee is a reliable sign of sufficient hydration.

Build Hydration into Daily Routine: Make it a habit to have a glass of water when you wake up, before meals, and before bed.

Flavor Water with Natural Additions: Infuse water with slices of fruits, vegetables, or herbs for added flavor. This can make hydration more enjoyable.

Alternate with Hydrating Foods: Incorporate foods with high water content, like cucumbers, watermelon, celery, and tomatoes, into your diet.

Consume Electrolyte-Rich Drinks: After intense exercise or in hot weather, consider replenishing electrolytes with sports drinks or natural alternatives like coconut water.

Incorporating Hydrating Foods and Beverages

Your total level of hydration can be increased by include foods and drinks that are high in moisture in your diet. Here are a few instances:

Cucumbers: A great snack to stay hydrated, as they contain approximately 95% water.

Watermelon: Packed full of vitamins and minerals, this fruit has one of the highest water contents, making it hydrating.

Coconut Water: After exercise, this naturally occurring, electrolyte-rich beverage can aid in restoring lost fluids.

Leafy Greens: Rich in water content, vegetables like kale, spinach, and lettuce are great additions to salads and smoothies.

Herbal Teas: Without adding extra calories or sugar, unsweetened herbal teas can help you meet your daily fluid needs.

Berries: Rich in vitamins and antioxidants, fruits like blueberries and strawberries also have a comparatively high water content.

Broths and Soups: Clear broths and soups made from vegetables can be a hydrating and nutritious addition to your diet.

Maintaining general health, promoting weight loss, and guaranteeing proper body functions all depend on drinking enough water.

SMART SNACKING

Eating small, healthful snacks throughout the day to help control blood sugar levels, increase metabolism, decrease appetite, and supply vital nutrients is known as smart snacking.

1. It reduces the need for insulin. Your blood sugar levels can be stabilized by eating small, healthful meals throughout the day. Avoiding overindulging in food during meals might be aided by doing this.

2. It Enhances metabolic process. You can increase your metabolism by eating small meals and snacks throughout the day. It follows that when you are at rest, your body expels more calories.

3. It Cuts down on appetite. You can maintain a feeling of fullness and satisfaction by eating healthful snacks. Your total calorie consumption may be decreased as a result.

4.It Supplies necessary nutrition. Eating nutritious snacks will assist you in obtaining the vital
 nutrients that your body needs. This can help to improve your overall health and well-being.

5. Healthy snacks are usually low in processed carbohydrates, sugar, and harmful fats and rich in protein and fiber.

Navigating Snacking for Weight Loss Success

A balanced diet should include snacks, especially for people trying to lose weight. When practiced consciously, it can aid in controlling hunger, supplying energy throughout meals, and avoiding overindulging. Here are some important things to think about:

Balanced Nutrition: Select snacks that provide a mix of macronutrients, such as complex carbohydrates, healthy fats, and protein. This gives you a feeling of fullness and continuous vitality.

Portion Control: Pay attention to serving sizes to prevent consuming too many calories. If not eaten in moderation, even healthful snacks might lead to an excess of calories.

Mindful Eating: Rather of eating out of boredom or stress, pay attention to hunger signs and eat when you're actually hungry.

Choose Nutrient-Dense Options: Opt for whole, minimally processed foods like fruits, vegetables, nuts, seeds, and lean proteins. These provide essential nutrients and help maintain overall health.

Healthy Snack Options and Portion Control

Here are some healthy snack options along with tips for portion control:

Mixed Nuts: A small handful of unsalted nuts provides healthy fats, protein, and fiber. Be mindful of portion size, as nuts are calorie-dense.

Greek Yogurt with Berries: Greek yogurt is high in protein and probiotics, while berries offer antioxidants and fiber. Stick to a recommended serving size for portion control.

Hummus with Veggie Sticks: Hummus is a good source of protein and healthy fats, and paired with veggie sticks, it makes for a satisfying and nutrient-dense snack.

Hard-Boiled Eggs: Eggs are a protein-rich option that can help keep you feeling full. One or two hard-boiled eggs make for a balanced snack.

Apple Slices with Almond Butter: This combination offers a balance of carbohydrates, healthy fats, and protein. Use a measured amount of almond butter for portion control.

Air-Popped Popcorn: Popcorn is a whole grain option that can be a satisfying snack. Use portion control and avoid excessive butter or salt.

Overcoming Emotional Eating Triggers

Snacking can provide a common difficulty in the form of emotional eating. The following techniques can help you avoid emotional eating triggers:

Identify Triggers: Note the circumstances, feelings, or happenings that frequently lead to emotional eating. Developing this awareness is the first step in changing for the better.

Find Alternative Coping Mechanisms: Take into account different coping mechanisms, like as journaling, taking a walk, meditating, or taking up a hobby, as an alternative to eating to deal with emotions.

Practice Mindfulness: Take a moment to check in with yourself before reaching for a food. Do you eat because you're physically hungry or because you're upset? You are able to make a more deliberate decision during this interval.

Create a Supportive Environment: Reduce the amount of enticing, less-nutritious meals in your immediate surroundings and surround yourself with wholesome snack options.

Seek Professional Help if Needed: For advice and assistance, consider consulting a healthcare provider or mental health professional if emotional eating becomes a serious problem.

A balanced diet should include sensible snacking, especially for people who are trying to lose weight. You can take proactive steps to reach your health and wellness objectives by selecting nutrient-dense foods, controlling portion sizes, and being aware of emotional eating triggers. Recall that snacking ought to be a deliberate and thoughtful component of your overall diet strategy.

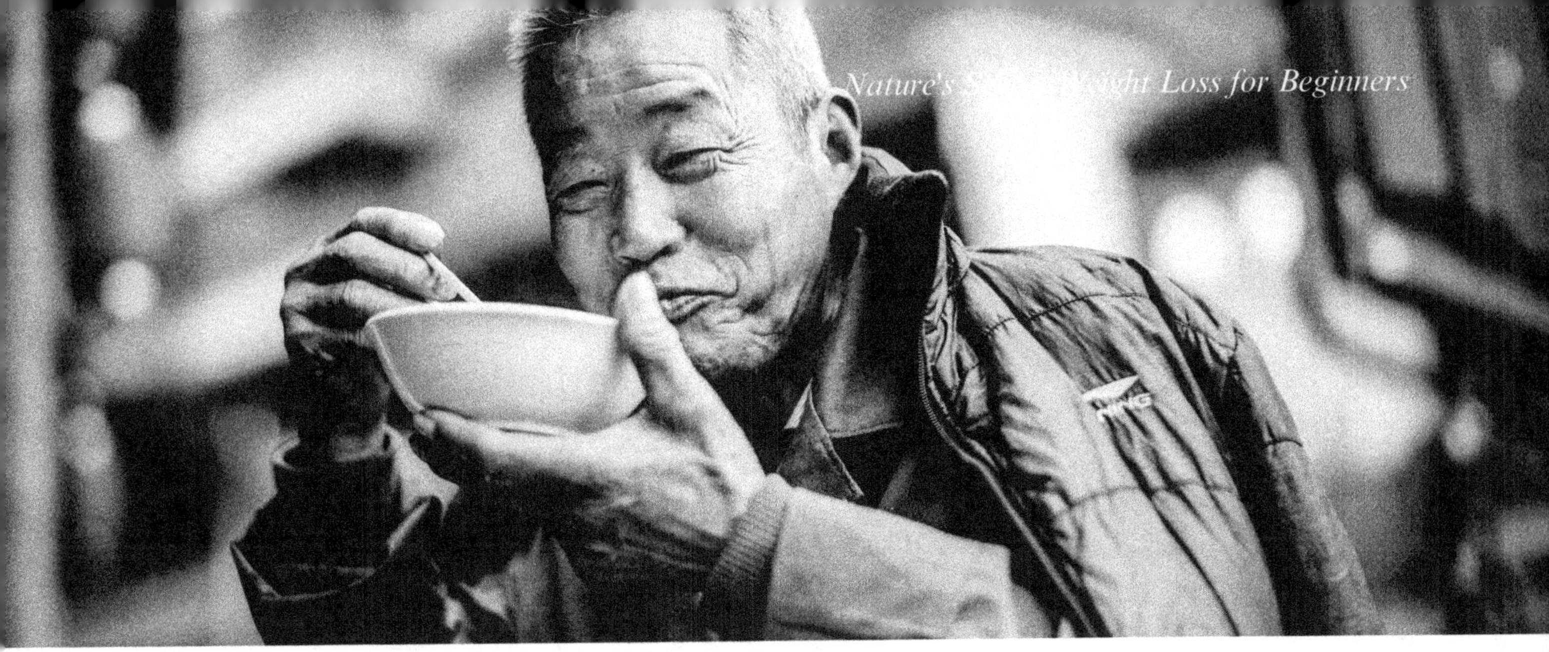

Eating Mindfully

What Is Mindful Eating?

In actuality, mindful eating is a method for controlling your eating patterns rather than a diet. You're encouraged to tune in, pay attention to your body's signals of hunger and fullness, and use your intuitive wisdom to establish an eating plan that works for you rather than adhering to rigid rules or tracking calories or points. Although this method can be difficult and even frightening at first, with practice you will be able to choose the kinds and quantities of food that will satisfy, nourish, and nurture you.

Weight loss is supported by mindful eating for a number of reasons. You must first distinguish between non-hunger cues that cause eating, such as seeing or smelling food or going through challenging emotions, and actual hunger, which is a physiological experience (for example, feeling lightheaded, dizzy, or low on energy). Thoughtfulness and the capacity to eat when you're hungry and quit when you're full replace automatic, mindless eating.

The Benefits of Mindful Eating for Weight Management

Eating mindfully entails paying close attention to what is being eaten as well as being completely present. It promotes observing indicators related to hunger and fullness as well as the tastes, textures, and experiences of food. The following are some advantages of mindful eating for controlling weight:

Enhanced Portion Management: Eating mindfully can help you become more aware of your body's hunger and fullness cues, which can
help you manage your portions and avoid overindulging.

Enhanced Knowledge of Food Selections: Mindfulness promotes a better understanding of the nutritional content of foods. This may result in more thoughtful and well-rounded eating selections.

Reduced Anxious Eating: Eating mindfully helps you become aware of your feelings and what makes you want to eat. This understanding can assist in ending the emotional eating pattern.

Savoring Food: By paying close attention to the taste, texture, and aroma of your food, you can derive greater satisfaction from each meal, potentially leading to fewer cravings for unhealthy options.

Improved Digestion: Eating mindfully promotes better digestion as you chew food more thoroughly, which aids in the breakdown of nutrients.

Techniques for Being Present at Meal Times

Being totally present when eating is a component of mindful eating. Here are several methods to assist you in doing this:

Eliminate Distractions: Put phones away, turn off displays, and establish a peaceful space devoid of outside distractions. This lets you concentrate only on your meal.

Use All Senses: Take full advantage of every sensation when dining. Take note of your food's flavors, textures, colors, and scents.

Eat Slowly and Chew Carefully: Savor each meal slowly. In addition to facilitating better digestion, chewing food completely lets you fully appreciate its flavor and texture.

In-Between Bite: Place your utensils on the ground in between bites. This allows you to take a time to listen to your body and determine whether you are still hungry

Recognizing Hunger and Fullness Cues

Developing an awareness of your body's signals of hunger and fullness is a cornerstone of mindful eating. How to identify these signals is as follows:

Hunger Cues:

- *physical Sensations*: Be aware of any bodily indicators of hunger, such as a rumbling stomach, dizziness, or a feeling of emptiness in your abdomen.

- *Heightened Awareness of* eating: The idea of eating becomes more alluring and alluring when you're truly hungry.

- *Consistent Energy Levels*: Eating when you're hungry contributes to a continuous supply of energy in the day.

Cues of Fullness:

- *Satisfaction and Contentment*: During your meal, take note of when you begin to feel full and content. This indicates that you are getting close to feeling full.

- *Slower Pace of Eating*: Often, fullness signals come on later than actual food intake. Eating gradually stops overeating by allowing these signals to catch up.

- *Diminished Interest in Food*: When you eat to fullness, you lose interest in it and may find the flavors less satisfying.

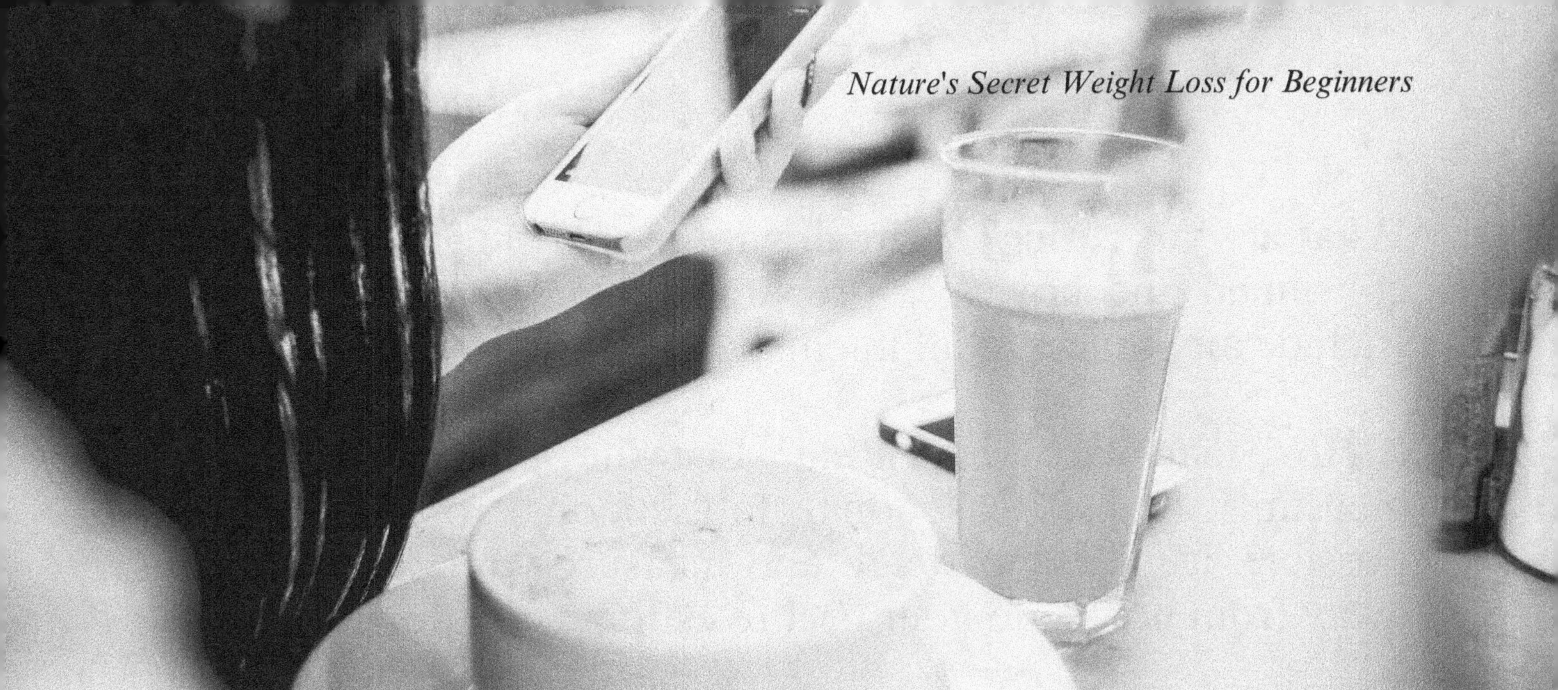

Tracking Your Food Intake

One helpful tool in this process is a food journal. It can assist you in recognizing the items, both healthy and unhealthy, that you frequently eat as well as in understanding your eating patterns and routines.
If you want to lose weight, the advise you'll get is to track what you eat. There are phone programs that integrate with fitness trackers and other devices to track anything from your workout regimen to your macros. Additionally, although keeping a food journal has its benefits, obsessing over every bite you take could have a negative impact on your emotional well-being.

What should you include in a food diary?

Accuracy and consistency are key components of a successful food journal, according to the majority of experts. What therefore ought to be recorded?
The following should be recorded in a basic food diary:

What are you eating? Write down the specific food and beverage consumed and how it is prepared (baked, broiled, fried, etc.). Include any sauces, condiments, dressings, or toppings.

...How much are you eating? List the amount in household measures (cups, teaspoons, tablespoons) or in ounces. If possible, it is best to weigh and measure your food. If you are away from home, do your best to estimate the portion.

When are you eating? Noting the time that you're eating can be very helpful in identifying potentially problematic times, such as late-night snacking.
Jotting down where you're eating, what else you're doing while you're eating, and how you're feeling while eating can help you understand some of your habits and offer additional insight.

Where are you eating? Record the specific place you are consuming food, whether it's at the kitchen table, in your bedroom, in the car, walking down the street, at a restaurant, or at a friend's home.

What else are you doing while eating? Are you on the computer, watching TV, or talking with a family member or a friend?
Who are you eating with? Are you eating with your spouse, children, friend, or a colleague, or are you alone?
How are you feeling as you're eating? Are you happy, sad, stressed, anxious, lonely, bored, tired?

The Value of Keeping a Food Journal

Keeping a food journal, whether in physical form or using digital tools, can be a powerful tool for promoting awareness of your dietary habits. Here are some benefits of maintaining a food journal:

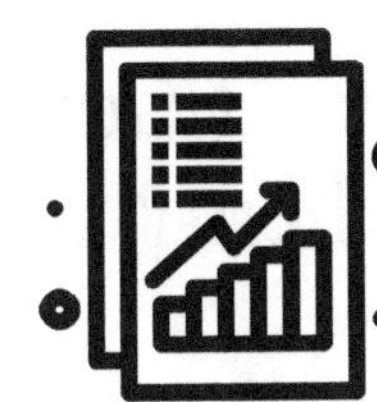 **Increased Awareness**: Writing down what you eat brings a level of conscious awareness to your dietary choices. It can help you notice eating patterns and make connections between your food choices and how you feel.

 **Accountability**: Recording your food intake provides a level of accountability. It can serve as a visual record of your dietary habits, making it easier to identify areas for improvement.

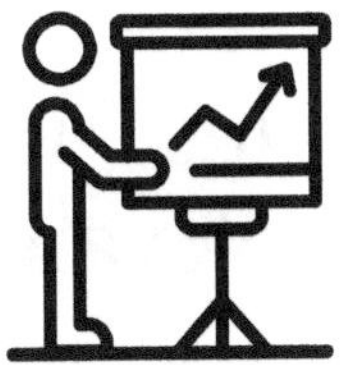 **Identifying Triggers**: A food journal can help you recognize emotional or situational triggers for certain eating habits. This awareness is a crucial step in making positive changes.

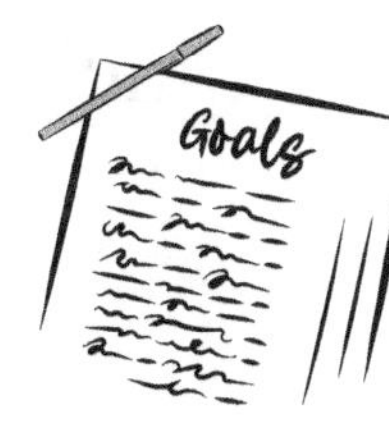 **Supporting Specific Goals**: Whether you're aiming for weight loss, muscle gain, or specific dietary changes, a food journal can help you track progress and adjust your approach accordingly.

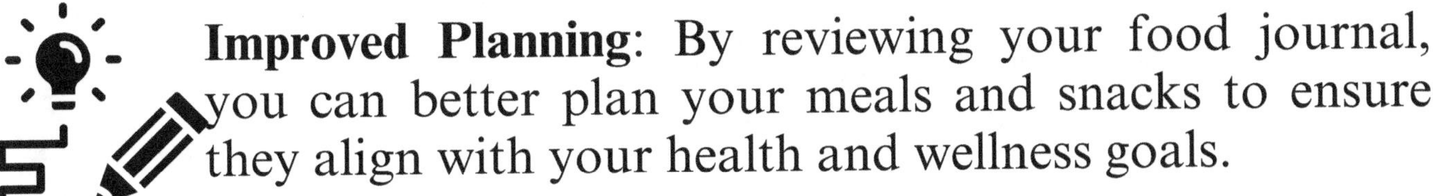 **Improved Planning**: By reviewing your food journal, you can better plan your meals and snacks to ensure they align with your health and wellness goals.

Tools and Apps for Monitoring Your Eating Habits

There are various tools and apps available that make it convenient to track your food intake. Here are some popular options:

MyFitnessPal: This app allows you to log your meals, track nutrients, set goals, and even scan barcodes for easy food entry.

Lose It!: Lose It! provides a comprehensive platform for tracking food, exercise, and weight loss progress. It also offers a barcode scanner and extensive food database.

Cronometer: This app focuses on detailed tracking of nutrient intake, making it a valuable tool for those interested in micronutrient balance.

Pen and Paper Journal: A physical journal can be just as effective. Simply record your meals, snacks, and any relevant details about your eating habits.

Photo Food Diary: Taking pictures of your meals can be a quick and visual way to track your food intake.

Analyzing Patterns and Making Informed Choices

Once you've tracked your food intake, it's important to analyze the data to make informed choices. Here's how:

 **Review Portion Sizes**: Ensure that you're accurately estimating portion sizes. This can be a key factor in understanding your overall calorie and nutrient intake.

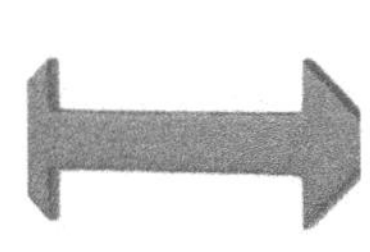 **Identify Nutrient Gaps**: Look for areas where you may be falling short on essential nutrients. This can guide you in making adjustments to your diet.

 **Notice Emotional Eating Patterns**: Pay attention to any patterns related to emotional eating. Are there specific situations or emotions that trigger certain eating habits?

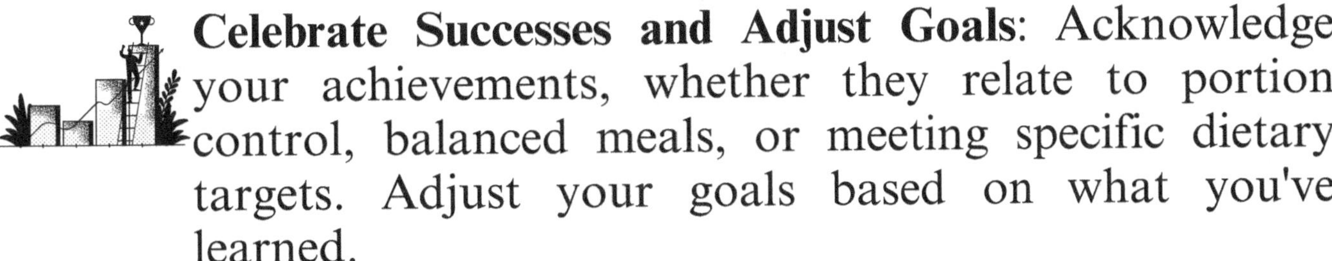 **Celebrate Successes and Adjust Goals**: Acknowledge your achievements, whether they relate to portion control, balanced meals, or meeting specific dietary targets. Adjust your goals based on what you've learned.

 **Seek Professional Guidance if Needed**: If you're struggling to make sense of your food journal or have specific dietary goals, consider consulting a registered dietitian or nutritionist for personalized guidance.

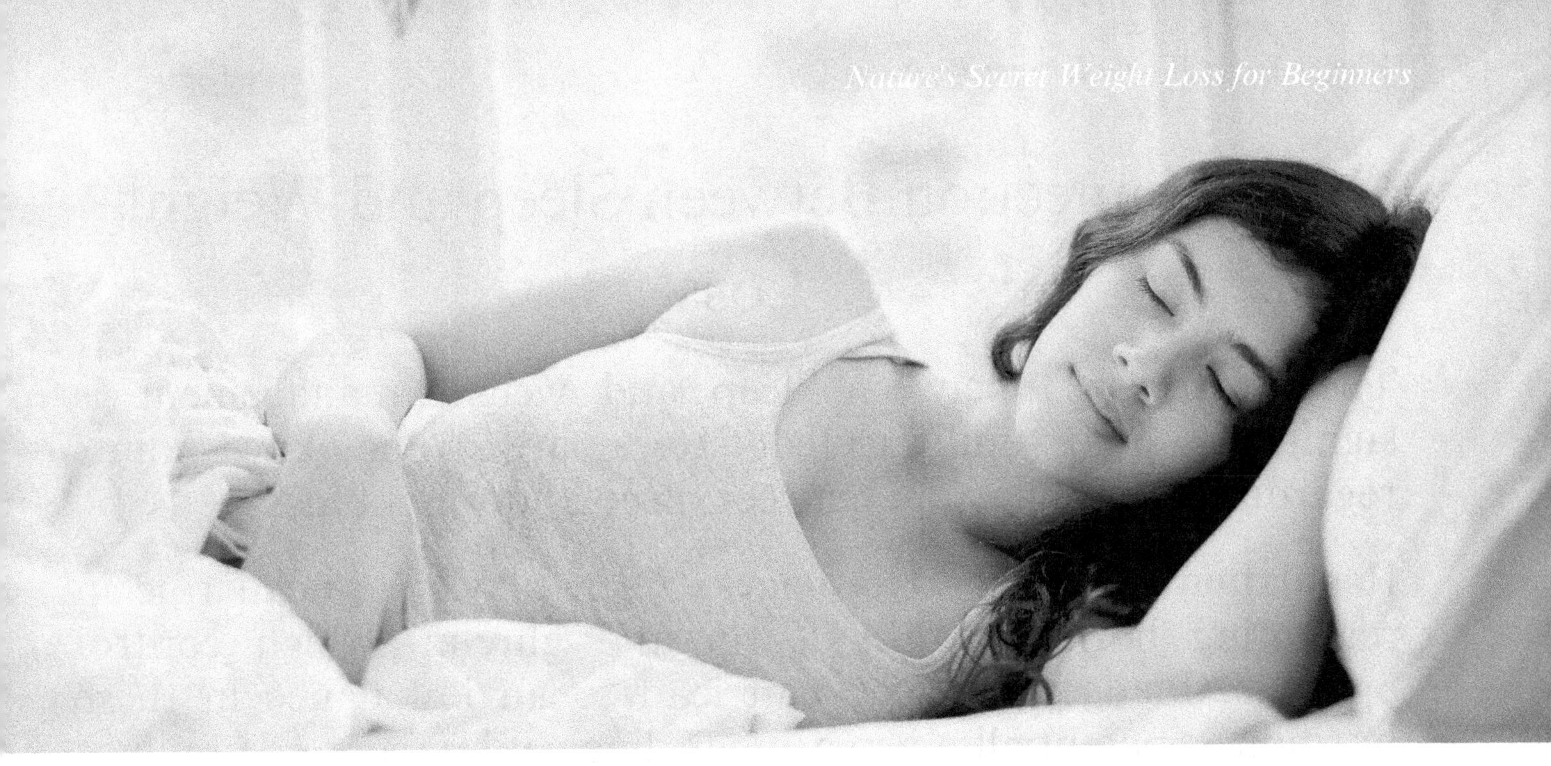

Getting Enough Sleep

Improved sleep lowers caloric consumption, which is revolutionary for weight loss plans.
Lack of sleep has a significant impact on weight. Your body was creating the ideal conditions for weight gain when you weren't sleeping.
It's simple to rely on a huge cappuccino to help you get going when you're sleep deprived. You might be tempted to order takeout for dinner because you're too tired to work out, skip the workout, and then arrive late because you're feeling uncomfortable. Sleep quality is just as crucial to your weight, health, and wellbeing as exercise and nutrition.

The Connection Between Sleep and Weight Loss

The relationship between sleep and weight management is significant and multifaceted. Here are some key points regarding the connection between sleep and weight loss:

Regulation of Hunger Hormones: Sleep plays a crucial role in regulating hormones like leptin and ghrelin, which control appetite. Inadequate sleep can lead to an imbalance in these hormones, potentially increasing feelings of hunger and cravings for high-calorie foods.

Metabolism and Energy Expenditure: Quality sleep supports metabolic processes. It influences how the body uses and stores energy, impacting overall calorie expenditure.

Regulation of Blood Sugar Levels: Adequate sleep helps regulate blood sugar levels, reducing the risk of insulin resistance and type 2 diabetes. Disrupted sleep patterns can lead to insulin sensitivity and weight gain.

Restoration and Recovery: During sleep, the body undergoes various processes of repair, recovery, and rejuvenation. This includes tissue repair, muscle growth, and the release of growth hormone, all of which are important for overall health and fitness.

Reduced Stress and Emotional Eating: Getting enough sleep can help regulate stress levels and mood, reducing the likelihood of turning to food for emotional comfort.

Strategies for Improving Sleep Quality and Duration

Improving sleep quality and duration is crucial for overall health and well-being. Here are some strategies to consider:

Establish a Consistent Sleep Schedule: Try to go to bed and wake up at the same time every day, even on weekends. Consistency helps regulate your body's internal clock.

Create a Comfortable Sleep Environment: Ensure your bedroom is conducive to sleep. This includes a comfortable mattress and pillows, appropriate room temperature, and minimal noise and light.

Limit Screen Time Before Bed: Avoid screens (phones, tablets, computers, TVs) at least an hour before bedtime. The blue light emitted from screens can interfere with melatonin production, a hormone that regulates sleep.

Limit Caffeine and Nicotine: Both caffeine and nicotine are stimulants that can interfere with sleep. Avoid consuming them in the hours leading up to bedtime.

Engage in Relaxation Techniques: Practice relaxation techniques such as deep breathing, meditation, or gentle stretching before bed to help calm the mind and prepare for sleep

Creating a Relaxing Bedtime Routine

A relaxing bedtime routine can signal to your body that it's time to wind down and prepare for sleep. Here are some calming activities you can include:

Reading or Light Stretching: Engage in low-key activities like reading a book or doing gentle stretches to relax your mind and body.

Mindfulness or Meditation: Practice mindfulness or meditation techniques to promote relaxation and calmness.

Aromatherapy: Use calming scents like lavender through essential oils, diffusers, or scented candles to create a soothing atmosphere.

Avoid Stimulating Activities: Steer clear of activities that are mentally or emotionally stimulating, as they can make it more difficult to wind down.

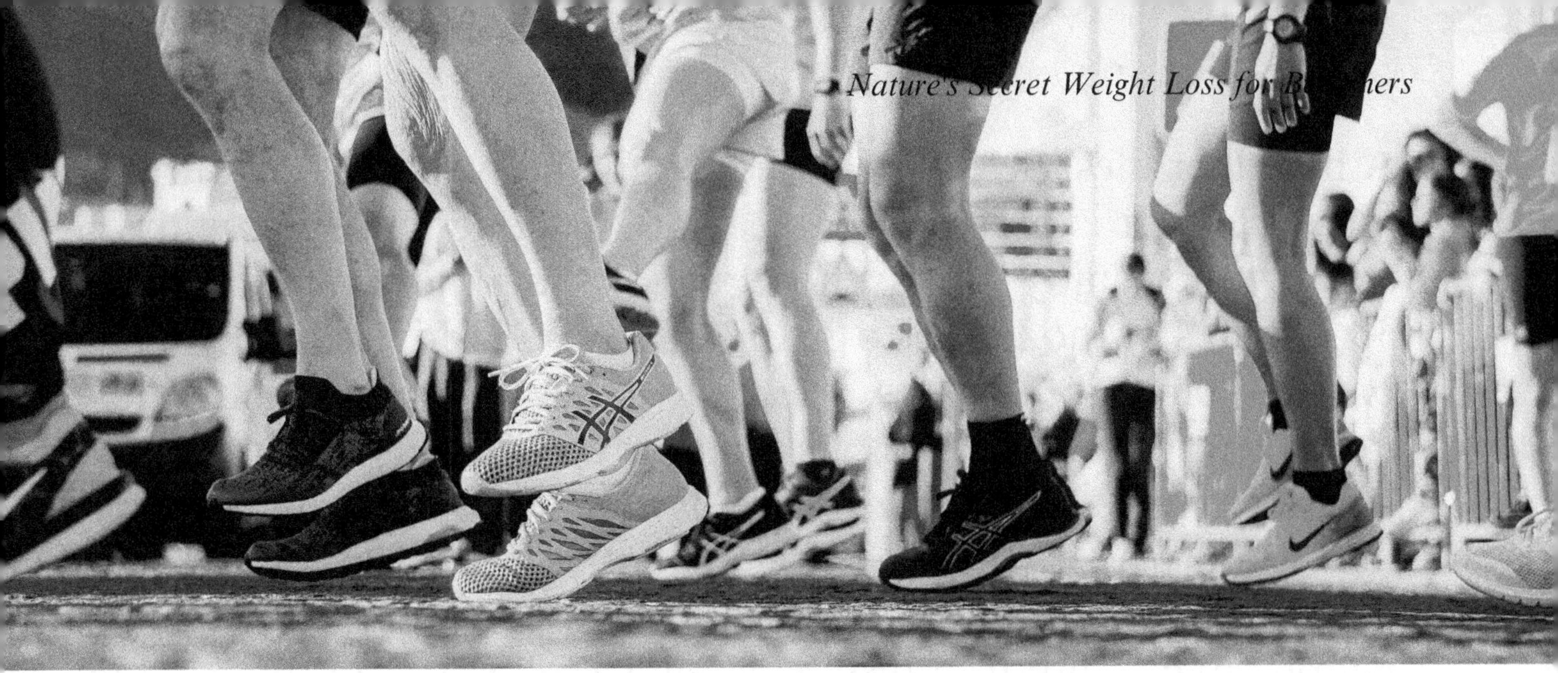

Exercising More Often

One of the seemingly endless advantages of exercise is that it can aid in weight loss. There are various ways that exercise aids in weight loss. Exercise is an essential component of any weight-loss plan since it burns calories, which is what you must do in order to meet your weight loss goals.

You will lose muscle and fat if you diet without exercising. Additionally, your metabolic rate may decrease when the percentage of muscle in your body decreases.
Exercise helps maintain a healthy metabolism, which helps it burn calories and not slow down too much when you cut back on food and drink.
Even in overweight people, physical activity can help reduce body fat percentage and thereby minimize their risk of heart disease. Additionally, exercise lowers stress levels. Regretfully, fewer than 5% of Americans engage in daily physical activity lasting thirty minutes.

A healthier lifestyle can be aided by any activity that encourages movement. It is more probable that someone will stick with an activity they enjoy if they chose it. For the majority of the week, 30 minutes of moderate-to-intense exercise is advised in order to prevent chronic diseases. Here is a list of some moderately intense physical activities. extending the activity's duration to 45–60 minutes at the most, is advised for maintaining weight loss. It may be beneficial to begin gently and work your way up to 45 or 60 minutes of physical exercise. Alternatively, some people may find it more beneficial to break up their daily activity into several 10-15 minute sessions.

Incorporating physical activity into your daily life

Incorporating physical activity into your daily life is essential for maintaining a healthy and active lifestyle. Here are some additional tips and strategies to seamlessly infuse exercise into your routine:

Active Transportation: Opt for walking or cycling whenever possible for short-distance trips. This not only adds physical activity to your day but also reduces your carbon footprint.

Take Active Breaks: Set regular reminders to stand up, stretch, and move around, especially if you have a sedentary job. Short, frequent breaks can help prevent stiffness and promote circulation.

Utilize Household Chores: Turn routine chores into mini workouts. Vacuuming, sweeping, gardening, and doing laundry all involve movements that engage various muscle groups.

Maximize Commuting Time: If possible, choose an active commute. If you use public transportation, consider getting off a stop early and walking the rest of the way. If you drive, park farther away from your destination and walk.

Stairs Over Elevators: Whenever you have the option, choose stairs over elevators or escalators. Climbing stairs is an excellent way to engage your leg muscles and get your heart rate up.

Incorporate Movement at Work: Integrate movement into your work routine. Consider using a standing desk, doing seated leg lifts, or incorporating desk stretches to keep your body active during the workday.

Engage in Active Hobbies: Pursue hobbies that involve physical activity, such as dancing, hiking, playing a sport, or practicing yoga. This way, you're enjoying yourself while staying active.

Make Playtime Active: If you have children or pets, engage in active play with them. This can be as simple as playing tag, going for a bike ride, or playing fetch with your dog.

Schedule Active Social Activities: Instead of meeting friends for coffee or a meal, suggest active outings like going for a hike, playing a sport together, or attending a dance class.

Utilize Technology: Use fitness apps or activity trackers to set goals, track your steps, and monitor your progress. These tools can provide motivation and help you stay accountable.

Embrace Household Fitness Equipment: If you have exercise equipment at home, like resistance bands, dumbbells, or a yoga mat, use them during free moments or while watching TV.

Finding Activities You Enjoy for Long-Term Commitment.

Finding activities that you genuinely enjoy is crucial for sustaining a long-term commitment to exercise.
Here are some additional tips and insights to help you discover activities that resonate with you:

Explore Varied Options: Don't limit yourself to one type of exercise. Try out a variety of activities, including different sports, fitness classes, outdoor adventures, and mind-body practices like yoga or Pilates.

Consider Your Preferences: Reflect on what you naturally gravitate towards. Do you prefer solitary activities like running or hiking, or do you thrive in group settings like team sports or fitness classes?

Tap into Childhood Passions: Think back to activities you enjoyed as a child. Whether it was dancing, cycling, or playing a specific sport, revisiting these interests can reignite your passion for movement.

Cater to Your Personality: Consider your personality traits. If you're competitive, you might enjoy sports or activities with a competitive edge. If you're more introspective, you might find solace in activities like yoga or tai chi.

Embrace Seasonal Activities: Take advantage of the changing seasons. Engage in winter sports like skiing or snowboarding in colder months, and opt for outdoor activities like hiking or swimming in warmer seasons.

Blend Fitness with Hobbies: Integrate exercise into existing hobbies. For example, if you enjoy nature, try hiking or birdwatching. If you're creative, consider dance, martial arts, or even circus arts like aerial silks.

Experiment with Classes and Workshops: Attend introductory classes or workshops in various activities. This provides a low-commitment way to explore new pursuits and see what resonates with you.

Listen to Your Body: Pay attention to how your body feels during and after different activities. Choose activities that leave you feeling energized, invigorated, and fulfilled, rather than drained or depleted.

Set Realistic Goals: Establish achievable goals based on your current fitness level and interests. This could be completing a 5k run, mastering a new yoga pose, or simply being consistent with your chosen activity.

Seek Social Connections: Consider activities that allow for social interaction. Joining a sports team, fitness class, or exercise group can not only make workouts more enjoyable but also provide a sense of community and camaraderie.

Be Open-Minded: Stay open to trying new things, even if they seem unconventional. You might discover a hidden talent or passion that brings a new dimension to your fitness routine.

Listen to Your Intuition: Trust your instincts when it comes to choosing activities. If something doesn't resonate with you, it's okay to explore other options until you find what truly sparks joy and enthusiasm.

Balancing Cardiovascular, Strength, and Flexibility Training

Cardiovascular Training:
- *Vary Cardio Activities:* Engage in a variety of cardiovascular exercises such as running, cycling, swimming, dancing, or using cardio machines. This keeps your workouts engaging and prevents plateaus.
- *Interval Training:* Incorporate intervals of high-intensity effort followed by periods of lower intensity or rest. This can enhance cardiovascular fitness and calorie burn.
- *Duration and Intensity*: Balance longer, steady-state cardio sessions with shorter, more intense workouts to challenge your cardiovascular system in different ways.

Strength Training:
- *Target Major Muscle Groups:* Include exercises that work all major muscle groups, including legs, chest, back, shoulders, and core. This promotes overall strength and balance.
- *Progressive Overload:* Gradually increase the resistance or weight you use for strength exercises to continuously challenge your muscles and stimulate growth.
- *Incorporate Compound Movements*: Compound exercises like squats, deadlifts, and bench presses engage multiple muscle groups simultaneously, providing efficient full-body workouts.

Flexibility and Mobility Training:
- *Include Stretching Exercises*: Regular stretching enhances flexibility and range of motion. Focus on both static stretches (holding a position) and dynamic stretches (moving through a range of motion).
- *Incorporate Yoga or Pilates:* These practices emphasize flexibility, balance, and core strength. They can be excellent complements to cardiovascular and strength training.

Guidance for Making Sustainable Lifestyle Changes

Setting Realistic Goals and Expectations

1.Define Specific, Measurable Goals (SMART Goals):
Specific: Clearly define what you want to achieve. Instead of "lose weight," specify "lose 10 pounds in the next three months."
Measurable: Ensure your goal is quantifiable. This allows you to track progress and celebrate achievements.

2. Consider Your Starting Point - Take an honest assessment of your current capabilities and lifestyle. This provides a realistic baseline from which to set your goals.

3. Break Down Larger Goals: - If you have a long-term goal, break it down into smaller, manageable milestones. Each milestone serves as a stepping stone toward your ultimate objective.
4. Set Timeframes: - Assign specific timeframes to your goals. This adds a sense of urgency and provides a clear deadline for achievement.

5. Prioritize Health Over Appearance: - Focus on goals related to health, well-being, and functionality rather than purely aesthetic outcomes. For example, aim to improve cardiovascular fitness or increase flexibility.

6. Consider Lifestyle and Commitments: - Ensure your goals align with your current responsibilities, schedule, and resources. Setting goals that are compatible with your lifestyle increases the likelihood of success.

7. Be Realistic About Rate of Progress: - Understand that progress may not always be linear. There may be periods of rapid improvement followed by plateaus. This is normal and part of the process.

Overcoming Challenges and Staying Motivated

1. Anticipate and Plan for Challenges:
- *Identify Potential Obstacles:* Consider what challenges you may face on your journey. These could be time constraints, work-related stress, or unexpected life events.
- *Develop Strategies:* Create a contingency plan for when challenges arise. This might involve having quick, healthy meals on hand for busy days or scheduling alternative workouts for days when your regular routine is disrupted.

2. Cultivate Resilience:
- *Shift Your Mindset:* View setbacks as opportunities for learning and growth rather than as failures. Recognize that progress is a journey, and bumps along the way are normal.
- *Practice Self-Compassion*: Be kind to yourself during difficult times. Treat yourself with the same understanding and encouragement you would offer to a friend.

3. Seek Support and Accountability:
- *Share Your Goals*: Confide in a trusted friend, family member, or mentor about your goals. Having someone to share your progress with provides a support system and can help keep you accountable.
- *Join a Community or Group:* Connect with like-minded individuals who are also pursuing similar goals. Online forums, local fitness groups, or classes can offer a sense of community and shared motivation.

4. Celebrate Small Wins: - *Acknowledge Achievements:* Recognize and celebrate even the smallest successes. Whether it's completing a workout, choosing a nutritious meal, or achieving a personal best, each accomplishment is a step forward.

Maintain a Progress Journal: Keep a record of your achievements, no matter how minor they may seem. Reflecting on your progress can boost confidence and motivation.

5. **Find Intrinsic Motivation**:

- *Reflect on Your Why*: Revisit the deeper reasons behind your desire for change. Whether it's improved health, increased energy, or setting a positive example for loved ones, understanding your intrinsic motivation can be a powerful driving force.

- *Visualize Your Success*: Imagine yourself accomplishing your goals. Visualizing success can reinforce your belief in your ability to achieve them.

6. **Incorporate Variety and Novelty**:

- *Change Up Your Routine*: Introduce new activities or workouts to prevent monotony and keep things fresh. Trying something new can reignite excitement and motivation.

- *Set New Challenges*: Continuously set and pursue new, attainable challenges. This could be increasing the intensity of your workouts, trying a different form of exercise, or setting a specific performance goal.

7. **Track Your Progress**:

- *Use Data and Measurements*: Keep records of your workouts, nutrition, and progress. Seeing tangible results, such as increased strength, improved endurance, or weight loss, can be highly motivating.

- *Regular Assessments**: Periodically evaluate your progress against your initial goals. This provides a clear picture of how far you've come and can renew your sense of purpose.

Nurturing a Positive Relationship with Your Body

1. Practice Self-Compassion

-Be *Kind to Yourself*: Treat yourself with the same kindness, empathy, and understanding that you would offer to a dear friend. Avoid self-criticism and negative self-talk.

- *Acknowledge Imperfections*: Embrace the fact that nobody is perfect, and imperfections are a natural part of being human. Celebrate your uniqueness and individuality.

2. Focus on Functional Health over Appearance:

- *Shift the Focus*: Instead of fixating solely on appearance-related goals, prioritize actions that promote overall health, vitality, and functionality.

- *Celebrate What Your Body Can Do*: Recognize and appreciate the incredible capabilities of your body. Whether it's dancing, lifting, running, or

simply breathing, each function is a testament to your body's resilience.

3. Practice Mindful Awareness:

- *Listen to Your Body*: Pay close attention to the signals your body sends. This includes hunger cues, energy levels, and signs of discomfort or fatigue.

- *Mindful Movement*: Engage in activities with awareness and presence. Whether it's yoga, tai chi, or simply walking, be fully present in the experience of movement.

4. Cultivate Gratitude and Appreciation:

- *Express Gratitude*: Take moments to express gratitude for your body. Reflect on all the ways it supports you, from carrying you through the day to allowing you to engage in activities you enjoy.

- *Practice Mirror Work*: Stand in front of a mirror and speak words of affirmation and gratitude to yourself. Acknowledge the parts of your body you appreciate and love.

5. Avoid Comparison and Negative Body Talk:
- *Limit Exposure to Unrealistic Images*: Be mindful of the media you consume. Avoid overly edited or unrealistic images that can contribute to feelings of inadequacy.

- *Challenge Negative Self-Talk*: When negative thoughts about your body arise, consciously replace them with positive affirmations or focus on the aspects you appreciate.

6. Surround Yourself with Positive Messages:
- *Curate a Positive Environment*: Surround yourself with messages, images, and people that promote body positivity and self-love. Follow accounts and communities that uplift and celebrate diverse bodies.

- *Diversify Your Influences*: Seek out diverse representations of beauty and body types in media and fashion. Exposing yourself to a range of bodies helps normalize and celebrate diversity.

7. Engage in Body-Positive Practices:
- *Body-Positive* Affirmations: Regularly repeat positive affirmations about your body. Affirmations

like "I love and accept my body just as it is" can reinforce a positive mindset.

Tracking Your Progress

The Importance of Monitoring and Celebrating Achievements

1. Provides Motivation and Encouragement:
- *Boosts Confidence*: Celebrating achievements reinforces your belief in your ability to make positive changes. It provides a confidence boost that propels you forward.

- *Fuels Intrinsic Motivation*: When you acknowledge and celebrate your accomplishments, you're more likely to be internally motivated to continue working towards your goals.

2. Offers Tangible Evidence of Progress:
- *Visual Confirmation*: Tracking and celebrating achievements provides concrete evidence that your efforts are paying off. This visual proof can be incredibly motivating.

- *Counters Discouragement*: In moments of doubt or when facing challenges, reflecting on past achievements serves as a reminder of what you're capable of achieving.

3. Reinforces Commitment and Accountability:
- *Affirms Commitment*: Celebrating achievements reinforces your commitment to your goals. It sends a message to yourself that you value and prioritize your health and well-being.

- *Holds You Accountable*: Regularly monitoring progress encourages accountability. It keeps you engaged and committed to the process.

4. Builds a Positive Feedback Loop:
- *Positive Reinforcement*: Celebrating achievements creates a positive feedback loop. You associate your efforts with positive outcomes, making you more likely to continue those efforts.

- *Stimulates a Growth Mindset*: Recognizing achievements fosters a growth mindset, where you view challenges as opportunities for learning and growth, rather than as obstacles.

5. Enhances Emotional Well-Being:
- *Boosts Mood*: Celebrating achievements releases feel-good chemicals in your brain, such as dopamine. This can lead to an improved mood and a greater sense of well-being.

- *Reduces Stress*: Taking the time to acknowledge your successes can help reduce stress levels and promote a more relaxed and positive outlook.

6. Maintains Perspective and Gratitude:
- *Prevents Negativity Bias*: During challenging times, it's easy to focus on setbacks. Celebrating achievements helps counteract negativity bias by highlighting the positives.

- *Fosters Gratitude*: Expressing gratitude for your achievements fosters a positive outlook and encourages a deeper appreciation for the progress you've made.

7. Strengthens Self-Efficacy:
- *Belief in Your Abilities*: Celebrating achievements reinforces your belief in your own capabilities. This sense of self-efficacy is crucial for maintaining confidence in your ability to reach your goals.

- *Encourages Taking on New Challenges*: When you see that you're capable of achieving one goal, you're more likely to take on new challenges and set higher aspirations.

Utilizing Metrics Beyond the Scale for a Comprehensive View

1. Body Measurements:
   - *Waist Circumference*: Measuring the circumference of your waist provides insight into changes in abdominal fat. A reduction in waist size can indicate progress, even if the scale doesn't show significant weight loss
   - *Hip Circumference:* Tracking changes in hip circumference can be important for assessing overall body composition and distribution of fat.
   - *Thigh, Arm, and Chest Circumference*: These measurements offer additional information about changes in muscle mass and body composition in different areas.

2. **Body Composition Analysis**:
   - *Body Fat Percentage*: Monitoring body fat percentage provides a more accurate reflection of changes in body composition compared to weight alone. It helps differentiate between fat loss and muscle gain.
   - *Lean Muscle Mass*: Tracking lean muscle mass indicates improvements in muscle tone and strength, which are essential for overall health and functional fitness.
   - *Visceral Fat Levels*: This measurement assesses the amount of fat stored around vital organs.
Reduced visceral fat is associated with lower risk of chronic diseases.

3. **Fitness Assessments**:
   - *Cardiovascular Endurance*: Evaluate your ability to perform cardiovascular activities over an extended period. This can be measured through activities like running, cycling, or swimming.
   - *Strength and Muscle Endurance:* Assessments of strength, such as lifting weights or performing bodyweight exercises, help gauge

improvements in muscular fitness.

- *Flexibility and Range of Motion*: Track improvements in flexibility, which are important for joint health and overall mobility.

4. Mental and Emotional Well-Being:

- *Mood and Stress Levels*: Keep a journal to note changes in mood, energy levels, and overall mental well-being. This provides valuable insight into the emotional benefits of your lifestyle changes.

- *Cognitive Function*: Pay attention to improvements in mental clarity, focus, and memory, which can be positively impacted by a healthy lifestyle.

5. Blood Markers and Health Indicators:

- *Blood Pressure*: Regular monitoring of blood pressure provides critical information about cardiovascular health.

- *Blood Sugar Levels*: Tracking blood glucose levels can be important for individuals managing diabetes or those looking to stabilize blood sugar for overall health.

- *Cholesterol Profile*: Monitoring cholesterol levels helps assess heart health and overall lipid profile.

6. Sleep Quality and Duration:

- *Sleep Patterns*: Keep a sleep journal to track the quality and duration of your sleep. Improved sleep is a key indicator of overall well-being.

- *Energy Levels and Alertness*: Note changes in daytime energy levels and alertness as indicators of improved sleep quality.

7. Nutritional and Dietary Metrics:

- *Food Intake and Nutrient Profiles*: Keeping a food journal or using a nutrition tracking app can help you assess your dietary choices and nutrient intake.

Conclusion

As you reach the end of "Nature's Secret Weight Loss for Beginners in 2023," take a moment to reflect on the incredible journey you've embarked upon. You've delved into the depths of natural and sustainable weight loss methods, uncovering the secrets that empower you to lead a healthier, more vibrant life. Along the way, you've gained invaluable insights and practical strategies that have the potential to transform not just your body, but your entire well-being.

Reflecting on Your Journey and Looking Ahead

As you reflect on your journey, remember that progress is a process, and every step you've taken is a testament to your dedication and determination. Whether you've made small changes or significant leaps, each effort has contributed to your overall growth and development. Take a moment to acknowledge and celebrate your achievements, no matter how modest they may seem. You are on a path of positive transformation, and every milestone is a cause for pride.

As you look ahead, envision the future you desire. Visualize the health, vitality, and well-being you aspire to. Know that you have the tools and knowledge to continue making informed choices that support your goals. Embrace the opportunities that lie ahead, and trust in your ability to overcome any challenges that may arise.

Encouragement and Final Words of Advice

In your pursuit of a healthier, more vibrant life, remember these key pieces of advice:

1. **Consistency is Key**: Small, consistent efforts lead to significant and sustainable change. Every positive choice you make contributes to your overall well-being.

2. **Listen to Your Body**: Your body is a wise guide. Pay attention to its signals and respond with kindness and respect. Nurture a relationship of trust and understanding.

3. **Celebrate Non-Scale Victories**: Remember that progress extends far beyond the number on the scale. Celebrate improved energy levels, increased strength, enhanced mental clarity, and all the non-physical benefits of your journey.

4. **Embrace the Journey**: This is not a race, but a journey of self-discovery and growth. Be patient with yourself, and enjoy the process of becoming the best version of you.

5. **Seek Support and Community**: You are not alone on this journey. Reach out to friends, family, or like-minded individuals for support, encouragement, and shared experiences.

6. **Stay Mindful and Present**: Cultivate mindfulness in your daily life. Be present in each moment,

whether it's savoring a nutritious meal, engaging in physical activity, or simply appreciating the gift of life.

7. **Believe in Yourself**: You possess incredible strength and resilience. Believe in your ability to overcome challenges and continue moving forward.

Wishing you health, happiness, and fulfillment,

[Author's Pen Name]
Janet R. Sheppard

Appendices

In this section, you'll find a wealth of additional resources, recipes, and tools to support you on your journey towards a healthier, more vibrant you. These resources have been curated to provide you with practical and actionable information, as well as delicious recipes to enhance your culinary experience.

1. **Additional Resources**:

   - Recommended Reading: A list of books, articles, and websites that delve deeper into the topics covered in this book. These resources provide further insights and perspectives on natural and sustainable weight loss.

   - Fitness Apps and Tools: A compilation of popular fitness apps and tools designed to help you track your progress, plan workouts, and stay motivated on your fitness journey.

   - Nutrition Guides: Access reputable sources for nutritional information, including guides on portion control, macronutrient ratios, and meal planning.

2. Recipes for Nourishment:

- Delicious Breakfast Ideas: A selection of nutritious and satisfying breakfast recipes to kickstart your day with energy and vitality.

- Wholesome Lunch and Dinner Options: Mouthwatering recipes that provide a balance of essential nutrients to fuel your body and support your weight loss goals.

- Snacks and Treats: Enjoyable and guilt-free snack options that satisfy cravings without compromising your commitment to a healthier lifestyle.

- Hydration-Boosting Beverages: Refreshing and hydrating drink recipes to complement your wellness journey.

- Mindfulness and Self-Care Exercises: Techniques and practices to promote mental well-being, reduce stress, and cultivate a positive mindset.

3. Additional Tips and Insights:

- Supplement Recommendations: Guidance on supplements that may complement your nutritional intake, along with tips on how to incorporate them safely.

- Mindful Eating Practices: Further techniques for practicing mindfulness during meals, fostering a deeper connection with the food you consume.

- Quick Reference Guides: Handy summaries of key concepts and practices covered in the book for easy reference.

These appendices serve as a valuable resource toolkit to support you in your ongoing journey towards a healthier and more vibrant lifestyle. Feel free to explore, experiment, and integrate these

resources into your daily routine as you continue to progress on your path to natural and sustainable weight loss.

Remember, every small step you take contributes to your overall well-being. Here's to your continued success and a future filled with health, happiness, and fulfillment!

[Author's Pen Name]
Janet R. Sheppard

FOOD TRACKER

DATE:

BREAKFAST

LUNCH

DINNER

WORKOUT

WATER INTAKE

NOTE